D0876052

MAYO CLINIC

5 STEPS TO CONTROLLING HIGH BLOOD PRESSURE

Sheldon G. Sheps

Medical Editor-in-Chief

Mayo Clinic
Rochester, Minnesota

5 Steps to Controlling High Blood Pressure provides reliable information on preventing and managing high blood pressure. Much of the information comes directly from the experience of health care professionals at Mayo Clinic. This book supplements the advice of your personal physician, whom you should consult for individual medical conditions. *5 Steps to Controlling Blood Pressure* does not endorse any company or product. MAYO, MAYO CLINIC, MAYO CLINIC HEALTH SOLUTIONS and the Mayo triple-shield logo are marks of Mayo Foundation for Medical Education and Research.

Published by Mayo Clinic Health Solutions

© 2008 Mayo Foundation for Medical Education and Research

All rights reserved. No part of this book may be reproduced or used in any form or by any means, electronic or mechanical, including photocopying and recording, or by any information storage and retrieval system, without permission in writing from the publisher, except by a reviewer, who may quote brief passages in review.

For bulk sales to employers, member groups and health-related companies, contact Mayo Clinic Health Solutions, 200 First Street S.W., Rochester, MN, 55905, or send an e-mail to *SpecialSalesMayoBooks@Mayo.edu.*

Address inquiries to Mayo Clinic Health Solutions, Permissions Department, 200 First Street, S.W., Fifth floor Centerplace Building, Rochester, MN, 55905

Stock photography from Artville, BananaStock, Brand X Pictures, Comstock, Corbis, Creatas, Digital Stock, Digital Vision, EyeWire, Food Shapes, Image Ideas, PhotoAlto, Photodisc, Rubberball and Stockbyte. The individuals pictured are models, and the photos are used for illustrative purposes only. There's no correlation between the individuals portrayed and the conditions or subjects being discussed.

Library of Congress Control Number: 2007938953

Printed in Canada

First edition

3 4 5 6 7 8 9 10

About Mayo Clinic

Mayo Clinic evolved from the frontier practice of Dr. William Worrall Mayo and the partnership of his two sons, William J. and Charles H. Mayo, in the early 1900s. Pressed by the demands of their busy practice in Rochester, Minn., the Mayo brothers invited other physicians to join them, pioneering the private group practice of medicine. Today, with more than 2,000 physicians and scientists at three major locations in Rochester, Minn., Jacksonville, Fla., and Scottsdale, Ariz., Mayo Clinic is dedicated to providing comprehensive diagnoses, accurate answers, and effective treatments.

With this depth of medical knowledge, experience and expertise, Mayo Clinic occupies an unparalleled position as a health information resource. Since 1983, Mayo Clinic has published reliable health information for millions of consumers through a variety of award-winning newsletters, books and online services. Revenue from these publishing activities supports Mayo Clinic programs, including medical education and medical research.

Preface

High blood pressure is a serious problem. Many of the 65 million Americans who have the condition are unaware that they have it, and only about 30 percent are taking steps to treat it. Approximately 70 million Americans are classified as prehypertensive, which means they have above-normal blood pressure that puts them at increasingly greater risk of developing definite hypertension.

A primary goal of *5 Steps to Controlling High Blood Pressure* is to inform you about how high blood pressure develops, what puts you at risk, how it's diagnosed and how it's treated. You'll also learn how to reduce your risk of the many conditions associated with high blood pressure, such as coronary artery disease, heart failure, kidney failure, stroke and dementia. You'll read about the proper use of medications, home monitoring and regular follow-up care. You'll also find the latest on issues of concern to women, children and special at-risk populations. All of this will help as you work with your doctor to make informed decisions regarding your health care.

5 Steps to Controlling High Blood Pressure focuses on the central role you play in a treatment program. It highlights five fundamental elements of a program: What you eat, how active you are, your use of tobacco and alcohol, how you manage stress, and how well you take medications. Separately, each step can improve your overall health and lower your blood pressure. When combined, the steps form a personalized program suited to your needs.

High blood pressure can almost always be successfully managed. This book, along with the advice of your personal physician, can assist you in living a longer, healthier life.

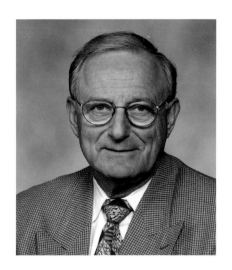

Sheldon G. Sheps, M.D.
Medical editor-in-chief

Editorial staff

Medical Editor-in-Chief
Sheldon G. Sheps

Managing Editor
Kevin Kaufman

Publisher
Sara Gilliland

Editor-in-Chief, Books and Newsletters
Christopher Frye

Contributing Editors and Reviewers
Brent Bauer, M.D.
Robert Brown, M.D.
Helmut Buettner, M.D.
Maria Collazo-Clavell, M.D.
Carl Cramer, II, M.D.
John Graves, M.D.
Donald Hensrud, M.D.
Richard Hurt, M.D.
Todd Johnson, Pharm.D.
Nancy Kaufman, R.D., M.P.H.
Edward Laskowski, M.D.
Carol Nash, R.N.
Jennifer K. Nelson, R.D.
Gary Schwartz, M.D.
Virend Somers, M.D., Ph.D.
Sandra Taler, M.D.
Stephen Turner, M.D.

Creative Director
Daniel Brevick

Art Director
Stewart Koski

Illustration
John Hagen
Michael King
Kent McDaniel
Chris Srnka

Photography
Richard Madsen
Jay Rostvold

Research Manager
Deirdre Herman

Research Librarian
Anthony Cook

Proofreading
Miranda Attlesey
Donna Hanson

Indexing
Steve Rath

Administrative Assistant
Beverly Steele

Table of contents

Part 2

Assess your health

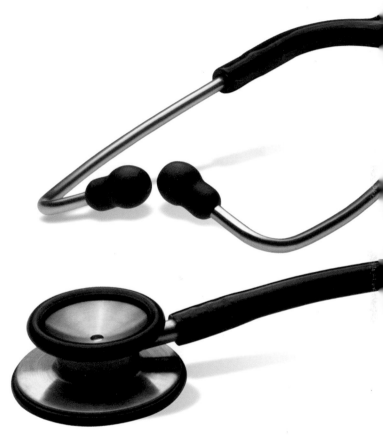

Contrary to what you may believe, you were not born to have high blood pressure. Your health is influenced as much by lifestyle as it is by genes. While family history is important, your weight, activity level, stress level and health habits play large roles in determining your future.

What this means is that your future isn't predestined. You can be in the driver's seat — you can play a vital role in managing your blood pressure and your overall health. The sooner you commit yourself to improving your lifestyle, the greater your chances of enjoying a long, productive life.

You may already be aware of some facts about high blood pressure. It's a common condition, especially among older adults. It's associated with other conditions such as stroke, heart attack, heart failure, kidney failure and forms of dementia. It's called the "silent killer" because it develops with no signs or symptoms — you may not be aware that you have the condition until after it has caused serious damage to your organs.

Here's something else that you should know: You can almost always control high blood pressure at levels that reduce your risk of serious cardiovascular disease. Medications are an important element of this control. But equally important is how well you take care of yourself. Weight, diet, exercise, tobacco and alcohol use, and stress are all aspects of your life that you can manage and try to change.

On the following pages are assessments to help you evaluate the health habits that most often influence your blood pressure: Are you physically fit? Are you eating well? Are you bothered by stress? Are you getting enough sleep? Keep in mind that good health is more than good physical health. It also includes good mental health. Mind and body are intricately intertwined — the state of one greatly influences that of the other.

Use the results from these assessments to identify general areas or specific

behaviors that you can work on to control your blood pressure and put you on the path to better overall health.

For example, you may find that you're getting enough physical activity but your diet could use a nutritional boost. Or you may feel that stress is preventing you from getting enough sleep.

The simple steps you take now to improve your health will, over time, turn into sustainable, healthy behaviors that can improve your nutrition and level of physical activity, as well as lower your blood pressure. Not only can you reduce your risk of disease and illness, but you'll feel better and you'll look great!

An important note: Don't view these assessments as a substitute for seeing your doctor. Regular exams are important for tracking your progress, identifying problems, getting direction and coaching, and adjusting medications. For a complete health assessment, you need the expertise of a health care professional.

Good luck as you begin your lifelong journey to manage your blood pressure, and all the best as you step up to a healthy future.

Are you fit?

1 **Do you have enough energy to enjoy the leisure activities you like to do?**

① rarely, or never
② sometimes
③ always, or most of the time

2 **Do you have enough stamina and strength to carry out the daily tasks of your life?**

① rarely, or never
② sometimes
③ always, or most of the time

3 **Can you walk a mile without feeling winded or fatigued?**

① no
② sometimes
③ yes

4 **Can you climb two flights of stairs without feeling winded or fatigued?**

① no
② sometimes
③ yes

5 **Are you flexible enough to touch your toes?**

① no
② sometimes
③ yes

6 **Can you carry on a conversation while doing light to moderately intense activities, such as brisk walking?**

① no
② sometimes
③ yes

7 **About how many days a week do you spend doing at least 30 minutes of moderately vigorous activity, such as walking briskly or raking leaves?**

① two days or less
② three to four days
③ five to seven days

How did you score?

To the left of the answer you chose is a point value — 1, 2 or 3 points. Add up the points from your answers for your total score.

A: If your total score was 18 to 21 points, congratulations! You're well on your way to overall fitness.

B: If your score was 13 to 17 points, you're on the right track, but your activity level could use a little boost.

C: If your score was 7 to 12 points, it's time to put getting in shape at the top of your to-do list.

Are your weight and eating habits healthy?

1 How do you score on the BMI chart? (See pages 56-58.)

① obese
② underweight or overweight
③ healthy

2 What's your waist measurement? (See pages 58-59.)

① considerably more than the recommended measurement
② slightly above the recommended measurement
③ at or below the recommended measurement

3 Do you have a health condition that would improve if you lost weight?

① yes
② possibly
③ no

4 Do you eat for emotional reasons, such as when you feel anxious, depressed, stressed, angry or excited?

① always, or quite often
② sometimes
③ never, or infrequently

5 Do you sit down and eat three regularly scheduled meals?

① never, or infrequently
② sometimes
③ always, or most of the time

6 How long does it generally take you to eat a meal?

① five minutes or less
② between five and 20 minutes
③ 20 minutes or more

7 Do you snack a lot, or substitute snacks for meals?

① yes, or quite often
② occasionally
③ no, or infrequently

How did you score?

To the left of the answer you chose is a point value — 1, 2 or 3 points. Add up the points from your answers for your total score.

A: If your total score was 18 to 21 points, congratulations! Your weight and your eating habits appear to be healthy.

B: If your score was 13 to 17 points, you're on track but you may consider losing a few pounds and improving some of your eating habits.

C: If your score was 7 to 12 points, you need to make a healthy weight and better eating habits a priority.

Are you eating well?

1 **How many servings of fruits and vegetables do you eat in a typical day?**

① one to three, or none
② four to seven
③ eight or more

2 **At the dinner table, do you shake salt on food before tasting it?**

① almost always
② occasionally
③ no, I always taste it first

3 **When you shop for bread, pasta and rice, how often do you buy whole-grain versions?**

① never
② sometimes
③ always

4 **Which of the following are you most likely to use in cooking?**

① butter or margarine
② corn oil
③ canola or olive oil

5 **How often during a typical week do you eat out and order convenience foods made with meat and cheese?**

① four or more times
② two or three times
③ once a week or less

6 **How many times during a typical week do you eat a noon or evening meal that doesn't contain meat?**

① once or never
② two or three times
③ four or more times

7 **What kind of milk do you usually drink?**

① whole milk or none
② 1 percent or 2 percent
③ fat-free milk or soy milk

8 **What are you most likely to reach for when you're thirsty?**

① regular sweetened soda
② fruit juice
③ water or another calorie-free drink

How did you score?

To the left of the answer you chose is a point value — 1, 2 or 3 points. Add up the points from your answers for your total score.

A: If your total score was 21 to 24 points, congratulations! You're making good choices and eating healthy.

B: If your score was 15 to 20 points, you're on the right track but your daily menu could use a tuneup.

C: If your score was 8 to 14 points, you could use some fresh ideas about good food.

How are your other behaviors?

1 Do you smoke cigarettes, cigars or pipes or use snuff or chewing tobacco?

① yes
② very infrequently
③ no

2 Do you drink more than a moderate amount of alcohol? (A moderate amount is one drink a day for men age 65 and older and women and two drinks for men younger than 65.)

① yes, often
② sometimes
③ never, or infrequently

3 Do you see a health care professional for regular checkups?

① no
② sometimes
③ yes

4 Do you wake up multiple times during the night or snore while you're asleep?

① often
② occasionally
③ never, or infrequently

5 Do you often feel sleepy during the day and have trouble functioning because you're tired?

① often
② occasionally
③ never, or infrequently

6 How would you rate your ability to handle daily stress?

① poor
② fair
③ good

7 How often do you feel lonely, depressed or pessimistic about what's happening around you?

① often, or always
② occasionally
③ never, or infrequently

How did you score?

To the left of the answer you chose is a point value — 1, 2 or 3 points. Add up the points from your answers for your total score.

A: If your total score was 18 to 21 points, congratulations! You're making wise decisions regarding your health.

B: If your score was 13 to 17 points, you're on the right track, but there's room for improvement.

C: If your score was 7 to 12 points, your behaviors may be putting your health in jeopardy. Select areas where you can make improvements and try to work on them.

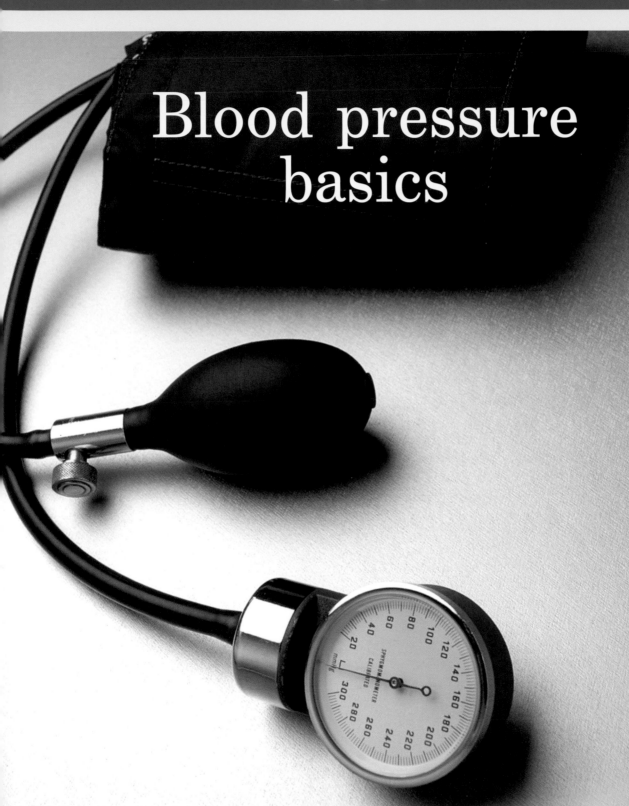

Part 1

Blood pressure basics

Chapter 1

What is high blood pressure?

If you're like many Americans, your blood pressure may be too high. Unfortunately, many people think that having high blood pressure isn't a big deal at all. But in fact, it is.

Left untreated, high blood pressure can cause your heart to work too hard and the walls of your arteries to harden, which impedes blood flow. It's one of the leading causes of disability or death due to stroke, heart attack, heart failure, kidney failure and dementia.

Fortunately, regular checkups, a good treatment plan and personal commitment can help you take control of the condition and reduce your risks of serious health complications.

Take the condition seriously

High blood pressure — also called hypertension — is the most common chronic illness in the United States. According to the National Heart, Lung, and Blood Institute (NHLBI), almost 65 million Americans have high blood pressure. That's about one out of every three adults. This total represents a 30 percent increase over the last decade in the number of adults with hypertension.

It's estimated that another 70 million American adults are designated with prehypertension. These individuals have a blood pressure level that falls just below the "high" category. Studies indicate that people with prehypertension are the ones most likely to develop persistent high blood pressure and serious cardiovascular complications.

High blood pressure isn't given the attention it deserves. It's often called the "silent killer" because many people affected by high blood pressure don't even know they have it. The disease generally doesn't produce signs and symptoms until it has progressed to an advanced stage. Of those with high blood pressure, about 70 percent are aware of their condition, but only 30 percent have taken steps to bring it under control.

"Control" means lowering your blood pressure to a level that reduces your risk of cardiovascular disease and other complications. But in controlling blood pressure, several factors may complicate the picture. One is age. People can develop high blood pressure at any age, but the risk increases as they grow older. According to the NHLBI's landmark Framingham Heart Study published in 2002, Americans who have normal blood pressure at age 55 still face a 90 percent lifetime risk of developing high blood pressure.

Another factor is race. About 29 percent of white Americans ages 18 and older have high blood pressure. Among blacks, the number jumps to about 39 percent. For Mexican-Americans, it's 28 percent, and this ethnic group has seen a sharp increase in the number of people with high blood pressure over the past decade.

Take the condition under your control

There's also plenty of good news to relate. High blood pressure doesn't have to be deadly or disabling. The condition is one of the most treatable forms of cardiovascular disease. If you know you have high blood pressure, there are steps you can take to lower it.

Keeping your blood pressure within a normal range for five or more years greatly reduces your risks of heart attack, stroke and kidney failure. That's where this book can help you. The chapters in Part 1 describe the basics of high blood pressure, with details on risk factors, screening and diagnosis.

Part 2 presents five specific steps you can take to control your blood pressure. The steps involve lifestyle changes and medications. Each chapter includes strategies that are simple and easy to follow. There's no strict regimens or numbers to keep track of. These are steps everyone can take. This information can help you get your blood pressure under control and guide you past obstacles that can easily derail your treatment program.

The first chapter in Part 3 informs you about treatment when you're at home or away from the doctor's office, including how to self-monitor your blood pressure, avoid drug interactions, and recognize an emergency. The second chapter focuses on high blood pressure in relation to specific groups, such as women and children, or to a concurrent condition, such as cardio-vascular disease or diabetes.

You can live long and live well after receiving a diagnosis of high blood pressure. But you have to be willing to do your part. The best course of treatment prescribed by your doctor is only as effective as your motivation to maintain the program. Whether your condition was recently diagnosed, you've had it for many years, or you simply want

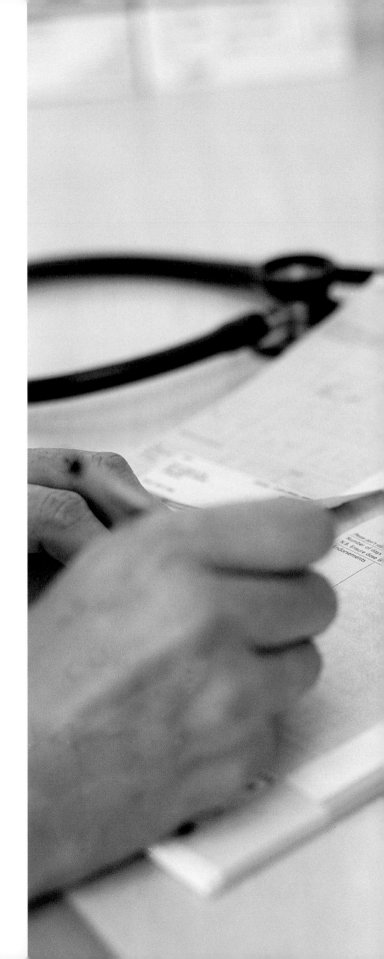

to prevent it, you'll find out how actions in your daily life affect blood pressure and learn ways to change bad habits into healthy ones.

Understanding blood pressure

To understand how high blood pressure develops and why it becomes so harmful to your health, it's useful to know some of the basics about your cardiovascular system and the organs that help to regulate it.

Cardiovascular system

Each beat of your heart releases a surge of nutrient- and oxygen-rich blood from your heart's main pumping chamber (left ventricle) into an intricate network of blood vessels (see illustration on page 21). Your arteries are the blood vessels that carry blood from your heart to the rest of your body. The largest artery, called the aorta, is connected to the left ventricle and serves as the main channel from your heart. The aorta branches into smaller arteries, which branch into even smaller arteries, called arterioles.

Microscopic vessels called capillaries carry blood from the arterioles into your body's tissues and organs. The capillaries exchange nutrients and fresh oxygen for carbon dioxide and other waste products produced by your cells. This oxygen-depleted blood returns to your heart through a system of blood vessels called veins.

When the blood in your veins reaches your heart, it's routed to your lungs, where it releases the carbon dioxide and picks up a new supply of oxygen. The freshly oxygenated blood is sent back to your heart, ready to resume the journey through your cardiovascular system. Other waste products are removed as your blood passes through your kidneys and liver.

A certain amount of pressure is required to maintain this circulation and keep all 11 pints of blood moving through your body. Your blood pressure is the amount of force exerted on your artery walls to keep the blood flowing continuously.

Blood pressure is often compared to the pressure inside a garden hose. Without an exerting force, the water can't get from one end of the hose to the other.

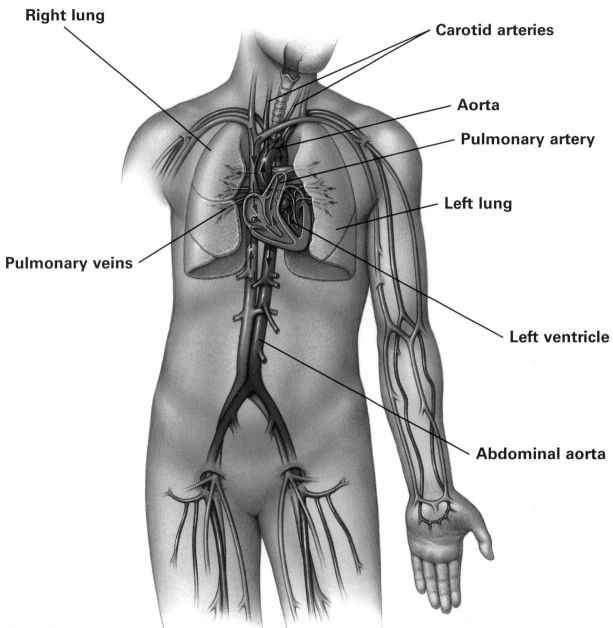

Right lung

Carotid arteries

Aorta

Pulmonary artery

Left lung

Pulmonary veins

Left ventricle

Abdominal aorta

Cardiovascular system

Each time your heart beats, blood is released from the left side of your heart (left ventricle) into the large blood vessel (aorta) that transports blood to your arteries (in red). Blood returns to your heart through your veins (in blue). Before being recirculated, the blood is sent to your lungs through the pulmonary artery to load up on fresh oxygen.

Regulators of blood pressure

Several organs and body chemicals work together to help control your blood pressure and keep it from rising too high or falling too low. They include your heart, arteries, kidneys, various hormones and enzymes, and your nervous system.

Your heart. The flow of blood in your body starts with your heart. When your heart releases blood from the left ventricle into your main artery (aorta), a certain amount of force is created by the pumping action of your heart muscle. The harder your heart muscle has to work to pump blood, the greater the force exerted on your arteries and the higher your blood pressure will rise.

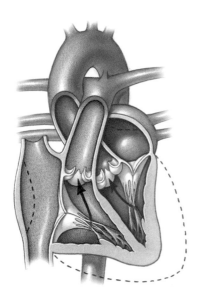

Systole (pumping)

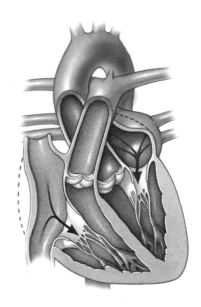

Diastole (resting)

Pumping action of the heart

During systole (left), your heart muscle squeezes blood out of your heart's pumping chambers (ventricles). Blood on the right side of your heart goes to your lungs, and blood on the left side is pumped into the large blood vessel (aorta) that feeds your arteries. During diastole (right), your heart muscle relaxes and expands to allow blood to flow into the pumping chambers from your heart's holding chambers (atria).

Your arteries. To accommodate the surge of blood coming from your heart, your arteries are lined with smooth muscles that allow the vessels to expand and contract as blood courses through them. The more elastic your arteries are, the less resistant they are to the flow of blood, and less force needs to be exerted by the heart on artery walls. When arteries lose their elasticity, resistance to blood flow increases and the heart has to pump harder. This increased force causes an increase in blood pressure.

Your kidneys. Your kidneys remove waste products from your blood and regulate levels of minerals such as sodium. The more sodium that's in your bloodstream, the more water that's retained. This extra fluid can increase blood pressure. In addition, too much sodium can cause your blood vessels to narrow, making the heart work harder and increasing pressure.

Other factors. Your central nervous system, along with body chemicals, also influences your blood pressure.

Baroreceptors. Within the walls of your heart and certain blood vessels are tiny node-like structures called baroreceptors. Similar to a thermostat that regulates the temperature of your house, baroreceptors monitor your blood pressure. If they sense a pressure change, they send signals to your brain to adjust your blood pressure to a normal range — which may involve slowing down or speeding up your heart rate or widening or narrowing your arteries. However, the "normal" range used by the baroreceptors is variable and can be reset in response to short-term changes in your blood pressure.

Epinephrine. Your brain acts on messages from baroreceptors by signaling the release of hormones and enzymes affecting the function of your heart, blood vessels and kidneys. One of the most important hormones to affect blood pressure is epinephrine (ep-ih-NEF-rin), also known as adrenaline.

Epinephrine causes your arteries to narrow and your heart to pump harder and more rapidly — both actions increasing the pressure exerted on your arteries. People often refer to the effect of epinephrine release as feeling pumped up or being on an adrenaline high. Epinephrine is released into your body during periods of high stress or tension, such as when you're frightened, in the midst of an argument or rushing to complete a task.

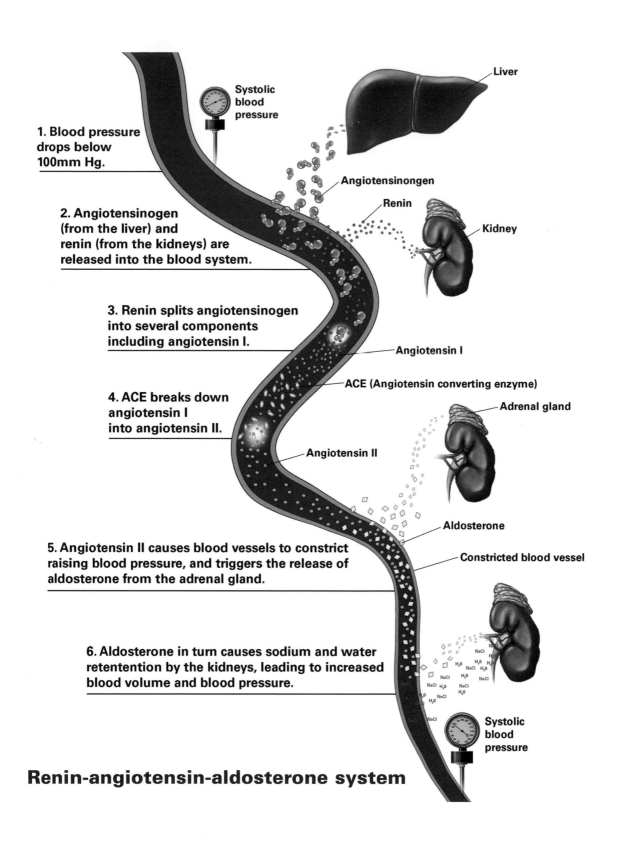

1. Blood pressure drops below 100mm Hg.

Systolic blood pressure

Liver

Angiotensinongen

Renin

Kidney

2. Angiotensinogen (from the liver) and renin (from the kidneys) are released into the blood system.

3. Renin splits angiotensinogen into several components including angiotensin I.

Angiotensin I

ACE (Angiotensin converting enzyme)

4. ACE breaks down angiotensin I into angiotensin II.

Adrenal gland

Angiotensin II

Aldosterone

Constricted blood vessel

5. Angiotensin II causes blood vessels to constrict raising blood pressure, and triggers the release of aldosterone from the adrenal gland.

6. Aldosterone in turn causes sodium and water retentention by the kidneys, leading to increased blood volume and blood pressure.

Systolic blood pressure

Renin-angiotensin-aldosterone system

The renin-angiotensin-aldosterone system. Your kidneys release the enzyme renin (RE-nin) into your bloodstream when blood pressure decreases. Renin works on the angiotensinogen protein, which triggers a complex process forming angiotensin (an-jee-o-TEN-sin) II. This substance constricts your blood vessels, increasing blood pressure (the process is illustrated on page 24).

Angiotensin II also stimulates release of a hormone called aldosterone (al-DOS-tuhr-ohn) from the adrenal glands located on top of your kidneys. Increased levels of aldosterone cause the kidneys to retain more sodium and water, also increasing pressure.

The effects of these compounds help the body make short-term adjustments to blood pressure, but these changes — which make the heart work harder — help lead to a gradual thickening of the heart muscle and blood vessel walls, leading to impaired function.

The endothelium. The walls of your arteries and veins are lined with an extremely thin layer of cells called the endothelium. This tissue layer plays a crucial role in regulating blood pressure by secreting chemicals that cause blood vessels to relax or contract.

For example, the endothelium contains nitric oxide that, when released, signals the smooth muscles in blood vessel walls to relax and expand, increasing blood flow and lowering pressure.

The endothelium also contains a protein called endothelin (en-do-THEE-lin), which acts as a potent vasoconstrictor. The narrowed vessel walls reduce blood flow and raise pressure.

What the numbers mean

An instrument called a sphygmomanometer (sfig-mo-muh-NOM-uh-tur) is used to measure blood pressure in your arteries. The device includes an inflatable cuff that's wrapped around your upper arm, air pump, and pressure gauge or digital meter. The cuff is inflated to squeeze the blood vessels in your arm. With a stethoscope, the doctor can listen to your pulse as the cuff is deflated, releasing the pressure on your blood vessels.

Blood pressure is expressed in terms of millimeters of mercury (mm Hg). The measurement refers to how high the pressure in your arteries is able to raise a column of mercury in the pressure gauge on a sphygmomanometer. Your blood pressure is usually based on the average of two or more readings taken when you're in a seated position and at each of two or more doctor visits.

Heart muscle contraction and relaxation

Two numbers are included in a blood pressure reading, and both are important. The first of the pair is your systolic (sis-TOL-ik) pressure. This is the amount of pressure in your arteries when your heart contracts — called systole (SIS-to-le) — and pumps blood into the aorta.

The second number is your diastolic (di-uh-STOL-ik) pressure. This is the amount of pressure that remains in your arteries between beats as your heart relaxes — called diastole (di-AS-to-le). Your heart muscle must relax fully before it contracts again. During this time, your blood pressure decreases until the next contraction.

The two numbers in a blood pressure reading are often written to look like a fraction. Systolic pressure is placed above or to the left and diastolic pressure is placed below or to the right. When stated verbally, the word *over* is generally used to separate the two numbers. For example, if your systolic pressure is 115 mm Hg and your diastolic pressure is 82 mm Hg, your blood pressure is written as 115/82, and spoken as 115 over 82.

In the first few months after birth, a baby's blood pressure is around 100/65 mm Hg, or 100 over 65. During childhood, pressure slowly increases. An ideal or normal blood pressure for an adult of any age is below 120/80 mm Hg. This is a reading you should always aim for, if possible. For certain individuals who are taking medication for high blood pressure, a blood pressure below 120/80 mm Hg may not be reasonable or tolerable.

Blood pressures between 120/80 and 139/89 mm Hg are classified as prehypertension. If you have prehypertension, it means your blood pressure is elevated above normal but hasn't yet entered the high blood pressure range — and yet you are at increased risk of cardiovascular disease, kidney disease and stroke. Having prehypertension should serve as a wake-up call, and your blood pressure should be regularly monitored as you try to control it.

High blood pressure is generally diagnosed in individuals with blood pressure that's 140/90 mm Hg and higher. As the table below indicates, blood pressure at 160/100 mm Hg represents a dividing line between stage 1 and stage 2 categories of hypertension.

Daily ups and downs

A single blood pressure reading reflects only what your pressure is at the moment it's measured. But throughout the day, your blood pressure naturally fluctuates. It increases during periods of activity when your heart works harder. And pressure decreases with rest or sleep when there's less demand on your heart. Your blood pressure also fluctuates with changes in body position, such as when you move from a lying or sitting position to a standing position. (See "When your blood pressure drops too low" on page 30.)

Classification of blood pressure

	Systolic (mm Hg**) (top number)		Diastolic (mm Hg) (bottom number)
Normal*	119 or lower	and	79 or lower
Prehypertension	120 to 139	or	80 to 89
Hypertension			
Stage 1†	140 to 159	or	90 to 99
Stage 2†	160 or higher	or	100 or higher

*Normal means the preferred range in terms of cardiovascular risk.

**Numbers are expressed in millimeters of mercury.

†Based on the average of two or more readings taken in a seated position, and taken at each of two or more visits. Systolic hypertension is a major risk factor for cardiovascular disease, even without elevated diastolic pressure, especially in older people.

Source: National Institutes of Health, 2003

Food, alcohol, pain, stress and strong emotions also increase your blood pressure. While you sleep, dreaming can raise your blood pressure. These ups and downs are perfectly normal changes in a typical day.

Your blood pressure even changes with the time of day. Pressure in your arteries follows natural fluctuations during a 24-hour period. It's usually at its highest in the morning hours after you awaken and become active. It generally stays at approximately the same level throughout the day and then late in the evening your blood pressure begins to decrease. It usually reaches its lowest level in the early morning hours while you're sleeping.

This 24-hour cycle is known as a circadian (sur-KAY-dee-un) rhythm. Your body has more than 100 different circadian rhythms, each influencing a different body function — for example, sleep patterns or body temperature.

If you're an evening or overnight shift worker, the circadian rhythm of your blood pressure differs from that of a day worker and is closely aligned to your schedule of work and rest. That's because many circadian rhythms change with altered patterns of activity.

Getting an accurate reading

To get a good indication of your average blood pressure, it's best to measure it during the day after you've been moderately active for a few hours. If you exercise in the morning, it's better to measure blood pressure beforehand. Following strenuous physical activity, blood pressure will fluctuate before readjusting to your average pressure.

You also shouldn't eat, smoke or drink caffeine or alcohol 30 minutes before measuring your blood pressure. Caffeine and tobacco can temporarily increase pressure. Alcohol may temporarily decrease it, although the opposite effect occurs in some people. Some over-the-counter medications, including decongestants, anti-inflammatory drugs and certain diet aids, can increase blood pressure for hours or even days after you take them.

In addition, you should wait five minutes after you sit down before taking a reading so that your blood pressure has time to adjust to your change in position and activity. Measuring your blood pressure under controlled conditions permits more accurate observations of how you're doing over time. If you have high blood pressure, your treatment plan might include measuring your blood pressure at home. See Chapter 4 for detailed instructions on home monitoring.

When pressure is persistently high

When the complex system regulating your blood pressure doesn't work as it's supposed to, too much pressure may build within your arteries. When increased pressure in your arteries continues on a persistent basis, it may be diagnosed as high blood pressure.

Hypertension is the medical term for this condition. Hypertension doesn't mean nervous tension, as many people believe. You can be a calm, relaxed person and still have high blood pressure.

Your blood pressure is considered high if your systolic pressure — the pressure when your heart contracts — is consistently 140 mm Hg or higher, your diastolic pressure — the pressure between heartbeats — is consistently 90 mm Hg or higher, or both.

In the past, doctors assumed that diastolic blood pressure was the best indicator of the health risks associated with high blood pressure. That's no longer strictly believed to be the case. While diastolic pressure remains an important indicator of risk for people under age 50, studies have shown that a high systolic reading is a serious warning sign of potential health risks, especially in older adults.

There are two separate stages of high blood pressure, based on increasing severity. They're referred to simply as stage 1 and stage 2. The terms *mild* and *moderate* are no longer used to describe stages of high blood pressure to avoid the possibility that people will mistakenly believe mild or moderate high blood pressure isn't serious.

High blood pressure generally develops slowly. Most often, people start out with normal blood pressure that progresses to prehypertension and, eventually, to stage 1 hypertension. Most people with uncontrolled high blood pressure are in stage 1.

Left untreated, high blood pressure can damage many of your body's organs and tissues. The higher the blood pressure and the longer it goes untreated,

When your blood pressure drops too low

Generally, the lower your blood pressure reading, the better. But in some cases, your blood pressure can drop too low, just as it can rise too high. Low blood pressure, called hypotension, can be life-threatening if it falls to dangerously low levels. However, this is rare.

Chronic low blood pressure — blood pressure that's below normal but not hazardously so — is fairly common. It can result from factors such as high blood pressure medications, complications of diabetes and the second trimester of pregnancy.

A potentially dangerous side effect of chronic low blood pressure is postural hypotension, a condition in which you feel dizzy or faint when you stand up too quickly. In the action of standing up, the force of gravity will cause blood to pool in your legs, producing a sudden drop in blood pressure.

Normally, your body counteracts a sudden pressure decrease by simultaneously narrowing your blood vessels and increasing the blood flow from your heart. When your blood pressure is chronically low, however, it takes longer for your body to respond to the change. Postural hypotension is more common with advanced age as nerve signals and regulatory system responses slow down.

You can often avoid this problem by standing up slowly and holding on to something while you stand. Wait a few seconds after standing and before you try to walk so that your body can adjust to the pressure change.

Some older adults, particularly those on medication for high blood pressure, may be at risk of fainting or falling after eating a meal. The cause can be a drop in blood pressure. If you've experienced falling or fainting after a meal, take preventive action by eating slowly and avoiding large meals. After you eat, rest for an hour.

See your doctor if you experience persistent dizziness or fainting. You may have another health condition that's causing the symptoms or that's making them worse than usual.

the greater the risk that damage will occur. Even stage 1 high blood pressure can be harmful if it continues over a period of several months to years. When this condition is coupled with other factors, such as diabetes, obesity or tobacco use, your risk of injury from high blood pressure increases.

Incidentally, it was conventional wisdom that an ideal systolic blood pressure was 100 plus your age. That's not true. Following this adage can deceive you into thinking that blood pressure at stage 1 or stage 2 levels is normal.

Signs and symptoms

High blood pressure is called the silent killer because it often doesn't produce any signs or symptoms.

Some people believe headaches, dizziness or nosebleeds are indications of high blood pressure. In fact, a few people may experience some nosebleeds or dizziness when their blood pressure rises. But a study has found no direct association between headaches and high blood pressure.

You can have high blood pressure for years without ever knowing it. The condition is most often discovered during routine physical examinations. Symptoms such as shortness of breath typically don't occur until high blood pressure has advanced to an extremely high — possibly life-threatening — stage. And even with very high blood pressure, some people experience no signs or symptoms.

Excessive perspiration, muscle cramps, frequent urination, and rapid or irregular heartbeats (palpitations) are sometimes associated with high blood pressure. But these signs and symptoms generally are caused by other conditions that can increase blood pressure.

Complications

High blood pressure needs to be controlled because, if ignored over time, excessive force on artery walls can seriously damage vital organs and tissues. The parts of your body typically affected by high blood pressure include arteries, heart, brain, kidneys and eyes (see illustration on page 32). Some complications may require emergency treatment.

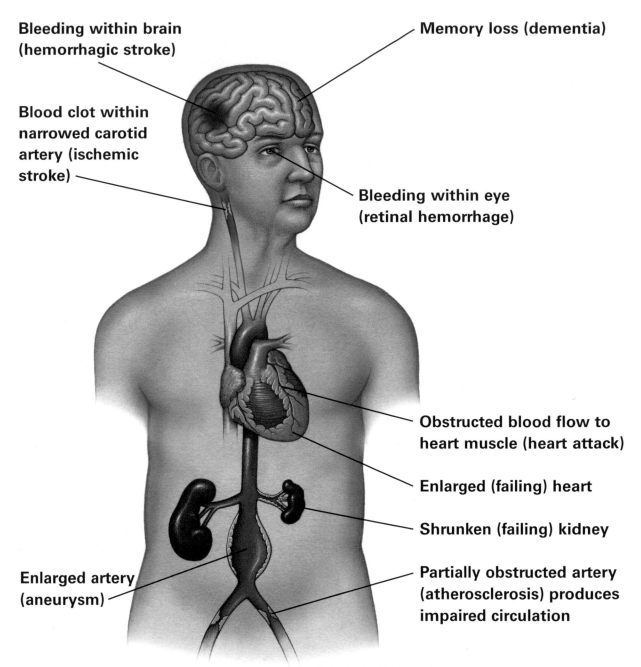

Bleeding within brain (hemorrhagic stroke)

Memory loss (dementia)

Blood clot within narrowed carotid artery (ischemic stroke)

Bleeding within eye (retinal hemorrhage)

Obstructed blood flow to heart muscle (heart attack)

Enlarged (failing) heart

Shrunken (failing) kidney

Enlarged artery (aneurysm)

Partially obstructed artery (atherosclerosis) produces impaired circulation

Complications of uncontrolled high blood pressure

Left untreated, high blood pressure can damage tissues and organs throughout your body. Sites in your body most affected by high blood pressure include your arteries, heart, brain, kidneys and eyes.

Damage to your cardiovascular system

Persistent high blood pressure creates a heavier workload for your heart and the network of arteries that carry blood throughout your body.

Arteriosclerosis. Healthy arteries are flexible, strong and elastic. Their inside lining is smooth, so blood can flow through them unrestricted. Over a period of years, too much pressure in your arteries can make the walls thick, stiff and less elastic, impeding blood flow. The term *arteriosclerosis* (ahr-teer-e-oh-skluh-RO-sis) comes from the Greek word *sklerosis*, meaning "hardening."

Atherosclerosis. High blood pressure accelerates the build up of fatty deposits in your arteries. *Ather-* in the term *atherosclerosis* (ath-ur-o-skluh-RO-sis) comes from the Greek word for "porridge," because the fatty deposits have a consistency of porridge.

When the inner wall of an artery is damaged, blood cells and fat cells often clump together at the injury site. They invade and scar deeper layers of the artery walls. Large accumulations of these fatty deposits are called plaques. Over time, the plaques harden.

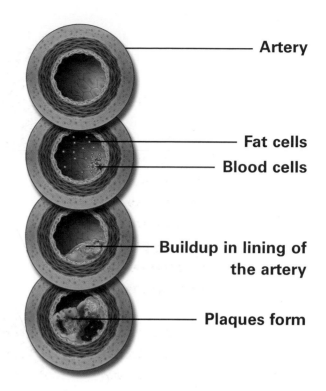

Artery

Fat cells

Blood cells

Buildup in lining of the artery

Plaques form

Atherosclerosis

The buildup of fatty deposits in your arteries leads to the formation of plaques, which can obstruct or block blood flow.

The greatest danger from the formation of plaques on your blood vessel walls is that organs and tissues served by these narrowed arteries don't get an adequate supply of blood. Your heart responds by increasing the pressure to maintain adequate blood flow. The increased pressure leads to further blood vessel damage.

Plaques may trigger the development of blood clots as blood flows past the blockage. Inflammation often occurs in areas around the plaques. Sometimes, the plaques break apart and the pieces combine with fresh blood clots to block the artery. Debris may also travel in your bloodstream until lodging in a smaller artery.

Arteriosclerosis and atherosclerosis can occur anywhere in your body but most often affect arteries in your heart, legs, brain, kidneys and abdominal aorta.

Aneurysm. When a blood vessel is damaged, part of the wall may bulge outward. This bulge is called an aneurysm. It commonly occurs in a brain artery or abdominal aorta (see page 73). If the aneurysm leaks or bursts, it can cause life-threatening internal bleeding.

In the early stages, aneurysms generally don't produce any symptoms. In more advanced stages, an aneurysm in a brain artery can lead to severe, persistent headache. An advanced abdominal aneurysm may cause constant pain in your abdomen or lower back. Occasionally, a blood clot lining the aneurysm wall breaks off and obstructs an artery downstream.

Coronary artery disease. The accumulation of plaques in the major arteries serving your heart, or coronary artery disease, is common among people with high blood pressure. If the heart muscle is deprived of too much blood, a heart attack may follow. The complications of coronary artery disease are the major cause of death in people with uncontrolled high blood pressure.

Reduced blood flow in the coronary arteries calls for an immediate trip to the emergency room and treatment with medication or angioplasty, a procedure for opening blood vessels.

Left ventricular hypertrophy. When your heart pumps blood into your aorta, it has to push the blood out against the pressure built up inside your arteries. The higher the pressure, the harder the heart has to work. And like any muscle, the harder your heart works, the larger it gets.

Eventually, the muscular wall of the heart's main pumping chamber starts to thicken (hypertrophy) from the excessive workload. The enlarged left ventricle needs an increased supply of blood. Because high blood pressure also causes the blood vessels feeding your heart to narrow, there's often an insufficient supply of blood to your heart. Controlling high blood pressure can prevent this hypertrophy.

Heart failure. Heart failure occurs when your heart doesn't pump effectively and is unable to circulate enough blood to meet your body's needs. As a result, fluid backs up and accumulates in your lungs, legs and other tissues, a condition called edema (uh-DEE-muh). The fluid in your lungs leads to shortness of breath. Fluid buildup in your legs causes swelling. Controlling high blood pressure can help reduce the risk of heart failure.

Your brain

High blood pressure increases your odds of having a stroke, also called a brain attack. A stroke is a type of brain injury caused by blocked or ruptured blood vessels that disrupt your brain's blood supply. Deprived of nutrients, the brain cells are damaged or die.

In results from the Framingham Heart Study, 56 percent of strokes in men and 66 percent in women were attributable to high blood pressure. The good news is that in people who were treated for high blood pressure, the stroke risk dropped by 42 percent over five years.

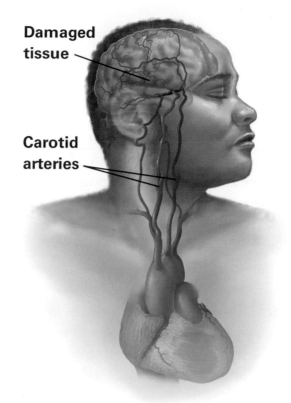

Damaged tissue

Carotid arteries

Ischemic stroke

When blood flow in an artery leading to the brain is obstructed, nerve cells are deprived of oxygen and nutrients. Brain tissue quickly may be damaged or die.

There are two basic types of stroke, characterized by the disturbance in the blood supply and by its location.

Ischemic strokes. Ischemic (is-KEM-ik) strokes are the most common type, accounting for about 80 percent of all strokes. Ischemic strokes usually affect the part of your brain called the cerebrum, which controls movement, language and the senses.

This type of stroke may result from a blood clot that has formed due to blockage from plaques. More than half of ischemic strokes are caused by stationary (thrombotic) clots that block an artery leading to your brain.

An ischemic stroke may also occur when a small piece of clotted blood breaks loose and is swept through larger arteries into smaller arteries in your brain. The moving (embolic) clot may become lodged and block blood flow, resulting in a stroke.

Sometimes, blood supply to the brain is briefly disrupted — for less than 24 hours. This occurrence is known as a transient ischemic attack (TIA), sometimes called a ministroke. A TIA is a warning sign of a possible stroke.

Hemorrhagic strokes. A hemorrhagic (hem-uh-RAJ-ik) stroke occurs when a blood vessel in the brain leaks or ruptures, usually caused by a development such as an aneurysm. Blood from the hemorrhage damages the surrounding brain tissue. And tissue over a broader area is damaged because it's deprived of blood. High blood pressure can predispose an individual to hemorrhagic stroke in the smaller arteries.

Improved detection and treatment of high blood pressure have contributed to a dramatic reduction in the number of strokes. When treatment lowers your blood pressure, your risk of stroke decreases remarkably — about 40 percent over a period of two to five years. Even if you've had a stroke or TIA, lowering your blood pressure can prevent these problems from recurring.

In addition, clot-busting medications given within the first few hours after an ischemic stroke begins can greatly reduce disability from the stroke.

Dementia. Studies suggest that damaged blood vessels in the brain caused by high blood pressure can lead to dementia, a progressive mental disorder that often includes memory loss, disorientation and personality change. The risk of dementia increases dramatically in people age 70 and older. After a diagnosis of high blood pressure, dementia can appear from a few years to several decades later. Recent evidence suggests that drug treatment to control high blood pressure may also lower the dementia risk.

Your kidneys

When blood circulates through your kidneys, the organs filter out waste products and regulate the balance of minerals, acids and fluids in blood. Each kidney contains over one million nephrons, which are tiny filtering systems consisting of small blood vessels and attached tubes. The kidneys help control blood pressure by regulating the levels of sodium and water. They also produce chemicals that control blood vessel size.

High blood pressure can interfere with these functions. Atherosclerosis due to high blood pressure can reduce blood flow to the kidneys, preventing them from eliminating enough waste from your bloodstream. The waste builds up and your kidneys may stop functioning, leading to kidney failure.

If your kidneys stop functioning, you'll need to undergo kidney dialysis, a process by which the waste products in blood are filtered out by machine, or you may need a kidney transplant.

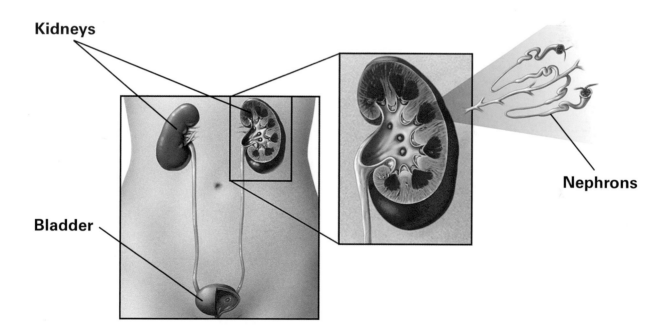

Kidneys

Bladder

Nephrons

How your kidneys work

Waste filtered from your blood by your kidneys is stored in your bladder as urine. Each kidney has more than a million nephrons that filter waste from the blood.

Your eyes

Occasionally, a simple eye exam leads to a diagnosis of hypertension because the small blood vessels of the retina are often the earliest and clearest indicators of high blood pressure. This condition is called hypertensive retinopathy.

In early stages, the tiny retinal arteries narrow. Eventually, the arterial walls thicken, compressing the adjacent veins and interfering with blood flow in the veins. Retinal blood vessels may tear or burst, leaking blood and fluid into the retinal tissue (see the image of retinal hemorrhage on page 72).

In severe cases of high blood pressure, fluid may also leak into the optic nerve, which causes swelling in the nerve (papilledema). Severe hemorrhaging in the retina and optic nerve leads to vision loss. Control of high blood pressure can almost always prevent these retinal complications.

Wrap-up

Key points to remember:
- Blood pressure is necessary for the continuous flow of blood that pulsates through your heart and blood vessels.
- High blood pressure means you have high readings on a persistent basis. That means systolic blood pressure that's consistently 140 millimeters of mercury (mm Hg) or higher, diastolic pressure that's consistently 90 mm Hg or higher, or both.
- High blood pressure typically doesn't produce any signs or symptoms.
- Left untreated, high blood pressure can lead to stroke, heart attack, heart and kidney failure, blindness, and dementia.
- By controlling high blood pressure, you significantly reduce your risk of disability or death related to the disease.

Chapter 2

Are you at risk?

With any disease, you naturally want to know its cause. Why does a condition occur in some people but not in others? Why does it develop in most adults after a certain age but for some people, the symptoms appear 10 or 20 years earlier? Unfortunately, the reasons why high blood pressure occurs in most people is unknown.

However, it's also clear that certain factors can put you at greater risk of high blood pressure. By knowing what these factors are, you can take steps to minimize the risk and possibly prevent or delay the disease from occurring.

To understand your risk, it's important to understand the two forms of high blood pressure — essential and second-

ary. Essential high blood pressure, also known as primary high blood pressure, is the most common form, estimated to occur in 90 percent to 95 percent of people with high blood pressure. Essential high blood pressure has no obvious cause, but certain genetic traits and lifestyle habits play important roles in its development.

In 5 percent to 10 percent of all blood pressure cases, a cause can be identified. This is called secondary high blood pressure because the condition is due to — or secondary to — another condition. Unlike the essential form, secondary high blood pressure may be correctable. When the underlying condition is treated, blood pressure may decrease or even return to normal.

Essential high blood pressure

Among a majority of Americans with high blood pressure, it's difficult to pinpoint exactly what's triggering the pressure increase. This condition is essential high blood pressure.

Genes may play an important role in the development of high blood pressure. But researchers are discovering a complex illness that typically doesn't follow the classic rules of genetic inheritance. Instead of stemming from a single defective gene, the condition appears to be a multifaceted disorder that, except in rare cases, involves interaction among several genes.

Essential high blood pressure results from a combination of various physiological factors related to:
- Motion (widening and narrowing) of your blood vessels
- Increased fluid in your blood
- Functioning of your blood flow sensors (baroreceptors)
- Production of chemicals that influence blood vessel function
- Secretion of hormones that affect your cardiovascular system
- Volume of blood pumped by your heart muscle
- Nerve control of your cardiovascular system

Risk factors such as weight, sodium use and physical activity also appear to interact with genetic factors. Generally, the more of these risk factors you have, the greater the odds that you'll have high blood pressure in your lifetime.

Risk factors you can't change

There are four major risk factors for high blood pressure that you can't change or control.

Race. Data from the Third National Health and Nutrition Examination Survey (NHANES III, updated 2007) show that high blood pressure occurs most frequently in the United States among black families that have been established in this country for generations. (There's still not enough evidence regarding black populations that have recently immigrated from Africa.)

The survey indicates that, among Americans age 18 and older, 39 percent of blacks versus 29 percent of whites have high blood pressure. The highest rates are among blacks living in the southeastern United States. High blood pressure in blacks generally develops at an earlier age than in whites. Plus, it's usually more severe and tends to progress more rapidly in blacks, leading to higher death rates from complications. According to the American Heart Association, hypertension may be a factor in 50 percent of all deaths in black men and 41 percent of deaths in black women with the disease.

Age. Your risk of high blood pressure increases with age. Although high blood pressure can occur at any age, it's most often detected in people age 45 and older. As noted in Chapter 1, Americans who have normal blood pressure at age 55 still have a 90 percent lifetime risk of developing high blood pressure.

It's fairly common for changes affecting your heart, blood vessels and hormones to occur naturally with age. These changes, coupled with other risk factors, may lead to the development of high blood pressure.

Family history. High blood pressure tends to run in families. If one of your parents has high blood pressure, you have about a 25 percent chance of

developing it during your lifetime. If both your mother and father have high blood pressure, you have about a 60 percent chance of acquiring it.

Just because high blood pressure exists in your family doesn't mean you're destined to get it. Even in families in which high blood pressure is prevalent, some members never develop the disease.

Sex. In the overall population of Americans age 20 and older, the prevalence of high blood pressure in men and women is roughly the same. However, among young and middle-aged adults, men are more likely to

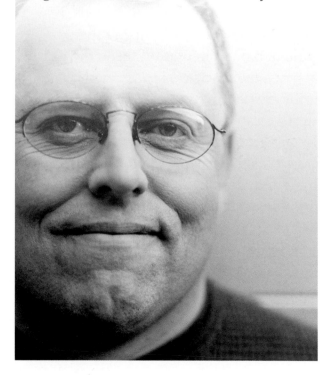

have high blood pressure than are women. After age 55, when most women are beyond menopause, the reverse is true. High blood pressure tends to be more common in women than in men.

Risk factors you can change

There also are many risk factors for high blood pressure that you can change and control.

Obesity. Being overweight increases your risk of high blood pressure for several reasons. The greater your body mass, the more blood you'll need to nourish your cells. Increasing the volume of blood circulating through your arteries requires your heart to pump with greater force.

Excess weight can increase your heart rate. It also increases the level of insulin in your blood, causing your body to retain more sodium and water.

In addition, some people who are overweight follow a diet that's too high in fat, especially saturated fat and trans fat. These fats promote atherosclerosis, causing your arteries to narrow. For most people, a diet contains too much

fat if more than 30 percent of total daily calories come from fat.

Inactivity. Lack of physical activity increases your risk of high blood pressure by increasing your risk of becoming overweight. People who are inactive also tend to have higher heart rates, and their heart muscle has to work harder with each contraction. The harder and more often your heart has to pump, the greater the force being exerted on your arteries.

Metabolic syndrome. This is a cluster of modifiable conditions that occur together — including high blood pressure, elevated blood sugar, excess body weight and abnormal cholesterol levels. These conditions make you more likely to develop diabetes, heart disease and stoke. The syndrome has also been called insulin resistance syndrome or syndrome X.

Although it's become a major health threat in the United States, metabolic syndrome often gets little attention. It's important not to ignore the risks. If you have all — or some — of the syndrome's components, take steps to reduce your risks of life-threatening illnesses. For more on metabolic syndrome, see pages 242-243.

The fattening of America

America's waistline continues to expand at an alarming rate. It's now esti-mated that 140 million adults are either overweight or obese. That's up from 97 million in the 1990s and represents nearly two-thirds of the adult popula-tion. Overweight is defined as having a body mass index (BMI) between 25 and 29.9. Obesity is defined as having a BMI of 30 or greater.

According to a report published in the April 5, 2006, issue of the *Journal of the American Medical Association*, comparing the years between 1999 and 2004, the rates of overweight and obesity increased for both sexes and across all races and ethnic and age groups. The report indicates that in 2003 and 2004, 66 percent of adults were overweight and 32 percent were obese. Those figures were up almost two percentage points from 1999 to 2000.

Adults aren't the only ones putting on excess weight. From 1999 to 2004, the prevalence of overweight among 12- to 19-year-olds rose more than two per-centage points to over 17 percent. The prevalence went from 15 percent to almost 19 percent for children ages 6 to 11 years, and from 10 percent to almost 14 percent for ages 2 to 5 years.

Problems with weight increase with age. The latest figures show that in 2004, 69 percent of women and 74 percent of men age 60 and over were over-weight or obese.

Excess weight is second only to smoking as a leading cause of preventable death in the United States. In 2000, about 400,000 U.S. deaths a year were associated with overweight or obesity. In comparison, 435,000 deaths a year were associated with cigarette smoking.

Tobacco use. The chemicals in tobacco can damage the lining of your artery walls, making them more prone to the buildup of plaques. Nicotine also makes your heart work harder by temporarily constricting your blood vessels, increasing heart rate and blood pressure. These effects occur because tobacco use triggers hormone production, including increased levels of epinephrine (adrenaline).

In addition, carbon monoxide in cigarette smoke replaces oxygen in your blood. This can increase blood pressure by forcing your heart to work harder supplying adequate oxygen to your body's cells. For details on stopping smoking, see Step 3 in this book.

Sodium sensitivity. Your body's cells need a certain amount of the essential mineral sodium in order to stay healthy. A common source of sodium is table salt (sodium chloride), which is composed of about 40 percent sodium and 60 percent chloride.

Some people are more sensitive to sodium in their bloodstream than are others. If you're sodium sensitive, you retain sodium more easily, leading to greater fluid retention and higher blood pressure.

It's estimated that up to 60 percent of Americans with high blood pressure are sodium sensitive. Among blacks, the percentage is even higher. Only about 15 percent to 25 percent of people without high blood pressure have sodium sensitivity. As you get older, your sensitivity to sodium often becomes more pronounced.

Unfortunately, sodium sensitivity is difficult to assess. Remember that most dietary salt comes as an added ingredient in foods, and since there's no health reason to consume excess salt,

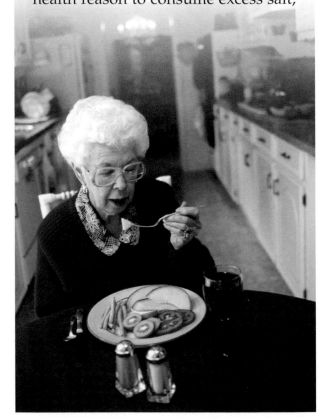

almost all of us can benefit from reducing sodium intake. For more on sodium intake, see Step 1 in this book.

Low potassium. Potassium is a mineral that helps balance the amount of sodium in your body's cells. It gets rid of excess sodium by way of your kidneys, which filter out the sodium that will be excreted in your urine. If your diet doesn't include enough potassium or your body isn't able to retain a proper amount, too much sodium can accumulate in your cells, increasing your risk of high blood pressure. For more on potassium, see Step 1 in this book.

Low potassium levels also stimulate the release of aldosterone, a hormone that increases retention of sodium and water, raising the risk of hypertension.

Alcohol consumption. Consuming three or more drinks of alcohol a day approximately doubles your risk of high blood pressure. How or why alcohol increases blood pressure isn't fully understood. But it's known that over time, heavy drinking can damage your heart and other organs.

The safest course is to drink moderately or not at all. For most men, moderate drinking means no more than two alcoholic drinks a day. For women, the limit is one drink daily.

Note that these are general recommendations for alcohol consumption, and individual guidelines may vary. For more on alcohol and high blood pressure, see Step 3 in this book.

Stress. High stress levels can lead to a temporary increase in blood pressure. If stress episodes occur often enough, they can damage your blood vessels, heart and kidneys. Results from the Coronary Artery Risk Development in Young Adults (CARDIA) study showed that participants with high levels of hostility and impatience had a significantly higher risk of developing persistent high blood pressure.

Stress can also promote unhealthy habits known to increase the risk of hypertension. For example, some people turn to smoking, drinking alcohol or overeating to relieve stress.

Other conditions

A chronic condition may put you at increased risk of developing high blood pressure or making it more difficult to control. Following describes several of these conditions.

In addition, women, children, older adults and people in certain ethnic groups may have specific concerns in controlling blood pressure. For details, see Chapter 5.

High cholesterol. High levels of cholesterol, a fat-like substance in your blood, promote the accumulation of plaques in your arteries (atherosclerosis), causing them to narrow and be too stiff to widen. These changes increase your blood pressure. See page 240.

Diabetes. Too much glucose in your blood can damage many of your organs and tissues, leading to atherosclerosis, kidney disease and coronary artery disease. These diseases all affect blood pressure. See pages 244-245.

Sleep apnea. Obstructive sleep apnea is a severe form of snoring that interrupts your breathing during sleep. Interrupted sleep can also be due to a disturbance in brain function. Studies have established a link between the interrupted breathing and onset of high blood pressure. For more on sleep apnea, see pages 245-246.

It's not always evident when you have sleep apnea. But if you consistently have trouble getting a restful night's sleep and have difficulty staying awake during the day, talk to your doctor. Being overweight or obese also contributes to the risk of sleep apnea.

Treatment may include losing weight, sleeping on your side rather than on your back, and using a mask device that gently blows air through your airway with just enough pressure to keep the passage open.

Chronic kidney failure. Kidney failure is both a cause and consequence of chronic high blood pressure. Added force on the tiny blood vessels within your kidneys can cause scarring and a slow, progressive loss of function. Your kidneys will no longer be able to filter waste, resulting in a buildup of waste and fluid in your blood. Chronic kidney failure can progress to a point where either dialysis or transplantation is the only treatment option available.

Heart failure. If your heart muscle is damaged or weakened, possibly due to a heart attack, it must work harder to pump blood. If you have uncontrolled high blood pressure, there's a much greater demand on your weakened heart. Over time, the heart muscle may become thicker to compensate for the extra work it must perform. Eventually, your heart muscle may become too stiff or weak to effectively pump blood. Heart failure means that your heart is unable to pump enough blood to meet your body's needs.

Other indicators for increased cardio-vascular risk include changes in the blood circulation of your retina, a thickening of the wall of the left ventricle — the main pumping chamber of your heart, changes in the level of creatinine (a waste product excreted by your kidneys) in your blood and the amount of protein in your urine. The treatment of high blood pressure often can slow or reverse the progression of these risk factors.

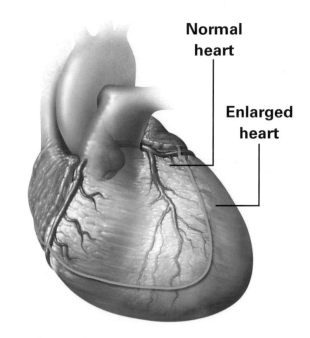

Normal heart

Enlarged heart

Heart failure

The heart may try to compensate for reduced pumping ability by getting larger.

A multiplying effect

Risk factors usually don't exist independently of each other and often interact. For example, if you're overweight and you're inactive, your odds of having high blood pressure are much higher than if you have either one of these factors alone.

By the same token, working to reduce one risk factor may have benefits for reducing the others. Your total reduction in risk may be more than the sum of that one factor alone.

Keep in mind: The word *risk* refers to your odds or chances — not to the inevitability of something occurring. Clearly, risk factors affect your chances of having high blood pressure, but having one or more risk factors is no guarantee of that happening. By the same token, you can develop high blood pressure even if you have no risk factors. The bottom line is that by reducing or controlling your modifiable risks factors, you lower your chance of getting the disease.

Secondary high blood pressure

The previous section has described essential high blood pressure as a condition likely caused by multiple factors, although the identity of each factor and the role it plays may be hard to define. With secondary high blood pressure, the condition is a direct result of another disorder.

Secondary high blood pressure usually has a more rapid onset and pushes blood pressure to higher levels than essential blood pressure does. When the underlying disease or condition is corrected, blood pressure typically decreases. In some people, blood pressure levels may return to normal.

Major causes

Secondary hypertension can be caused by a variety of conditions. Here are some of the primary causes.

Kidney problems. Kidneys are important regulators of blood pressure, and various kidney problems may account for a large number of secondary high blood pressure cases.

Kidney diseases such as polycystic kidneys — an inherited disorder, diabetic kidney disease, nephritis and scleroderma cause damage that can lead to kidney failure. When your kidneys can no longer get rid of sodium, water and waste products as they normally do, the scarring and narrowing of blood vessels that results can raise your blood pressure. Damaged kidneys also may release chemicals that raise your blood pressure (see pages 246-247).

If kidney disease is suspected, your doctor will perform a physical examination. Tests that detect elevated levels of waste products in your blood and excess protein in your urine may indicate kidney malfunction. Imaging tests such as ultrasound, computerized tomography (CT) or magnetic resonance imaging (MRI) can reveal cysts or scars caused by kidney disease.

In some cases, surgery may be necessary to reduce the number and size of cysts to help preserve functional kidney tissue. In severe cases, kidney transplantation may be required.

Obstruction of the renal artery. The renal artery is the main vessel supplying blood to each kidney. Obstruction is often due to a narrowing of the artery caused by atherosclerosis. When the obstruction is severe, the kidney may shrink and scar irreversibly.

Obstruction can also be caused by a condition called fibromuscular dysplasia. In this condition the middle layer of the artery wall (known as the media) thickens, narrowing the artery. The artery may have narrowed sections alternating with widened sections, which may form small aneurysms. One or both kidneys may be affected.

Narrowing of the arteries can impair kidney function and lead to the pro-

duction of a hormone that raises blood pressure. If this form of high blood pressure doesn't respond to drug treatment or if kidney function is severely impaired, the obstruction may be opened with catheters and stents similar to those used in treating narrowed coronary arteries.

Sometimes, narrowed renal arteries can be diagnosed with a stethoscope — the turbulent blood flow produces distinctive sounds. Narrowed arteries and changes in your kidneys can also be detected through imaging involving ultrasound, angiography, CT, MRI and nuclear scanning.

Pheochromocytoma. This condition occurs when a tumor forms in the inner layer of an adrenal gland. You have two adrenal glands, one atop each of your kidneys. The tumors, which can occur in other parts of your body and in multiple locations, secrete the hormones epinephrine and norepinephrine as well as other chemicals.

Pheochromocytoma almost always causes noticeable signs and symptoms. If you have one of these tumors, you may experience spells of sudden severe headache, heart palpitations and profuse perspiration, during which time

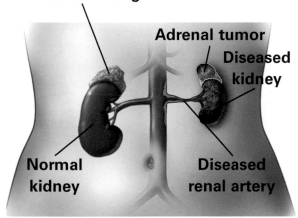

Normal adrenal gland

Adrenal tumor

Diseased kidney

Normal kidney

Diseased renal artery

Kidney problems

Among common causes of secondary hypertension are kidney disease, narrowing of the renal artery and a tumor in the adrenal gland (pheochromocytoma).

you appear pale. These spells may last from minutes to an hour. They may recur daily or infrequently. Your blood pressure is almost always markedly elevated during a spell, and may also be high between spells.

Diagnostic tests include blood and urine tests and imaging with CT, MRI or isotopes. Genetic tests also may be helpful, because this condition can run in families. The tumor is rarely malignant and can be removed by surgery.

Coarctation of the aorta. This condition involves a narrowing of the primary artery (aorta) from your heart. Coarctation usually occurs in the portion of the aorta located in your chest and rarely in your abdomen. It's usually detected at birth, but occasionally a person may reach adulthood before the condition is detected.

A narrowed aorta results in high blood pressure in your arms and low blood pressure in your legs. This can be detected when a doctor feels the artery in your groin and at your wrist simultaneously. The pulse in your groin will be slightly delayed and less forceful than the pulse at your wrist. A chest X-ray and imaging with ultrasound or MRI can establish the diagnosis.

Coarctation is repaired surgically by removing the narrowed portion of the aorta, and rejoining the ends of the vessel. In certain cases, for example if narrowing recurs after surgery, angioplasty is used to stretch open the narrow section using a balloon on the end of a catheter (balloon dilatation). If angioplasty fails to permanently expand the area, a metallic stent may be inserted through the catheter to hold the area open. While the long-term success of these stents is still unknown, the results so far are encouraging.

Thyroid dysfunction. The thyroid gland regulates your metabolism, from how fast your heart beats to how quickly you burn calories. As long as the gland produces the right amount of the hormone thyroxine, your metabolism functions normally. Sometimes the gland produces too much or too little thyroxine, upsetting the balance of chemical reactions in your body.

Hyperthyroidism. Overproduction of thyroxine may elevate your systolic blood pressure and heart rate. Signs and symptoms include:
- Nervousness
- Weight loss
- Excessive perspiration
- Prominent eyes (exophthalmos)

- Heat intolerance
- Palpitations
- Enlarged thyroid or presence of nodules on your thyroid
- Tremor
- Fatigue

Hyperthyroidism may run in families. Treatment, which can restore normal blood pressure, includes medication, radioactive iodine and, rarely, surgery.

Hypothyroidism. Underproduction of thyroxine also causes high blood pressure — both systolic and diastolic. Signs and symptoms include:
- Cold intolerance
- Coarse skin
- Fatigue
- Low, husky voice
- Slowing of body functions
- Puffiness of eyes, legs and hands
- Weight gain

This condition may occur after treatment of an overactive thyroid or inflammation of the thyroid gland. Treatment with thyroxine usually restores your body to normal.

Cushing's syndrome and aldosteronism. Cushing's syndrome is the result of excessive amounts of the hormone cortisol in your body. Cortisol can be produced by sources including the adrenal glands or come from medication such as prednisone. Adrenal gland disorders can run in families. Excess cortisol can cause physiological change or help cause disease, including:
- Increased fatty deposits on your face, neck and trunk
- Thinned skin, purple stretch marks, easy bruising and excessive hair growth
- Emotional instability
- Weight gain
- High blood pressure
- Weakness
- Diabetes
- Osteoporosis

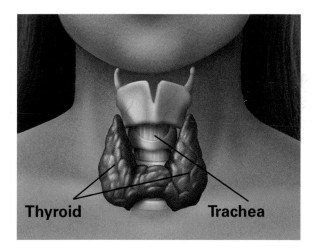

Thyroid gland
Abnormal hormone production in the butterfly-shaped thyroid gland can cause hyperthyroidism or hypothyroidism.

Treatment is directed at reducing the excess amounts of cortisol and can include eliminating or changing medications and having surgery if the problem is internal in origin.

Excessive secretion of aldosterone from your adrenal gland (aldosteronism) also can cause high blood pressure. Aldosterone causes your body to retain sodium and water and may also result in the loss of potassium by your kidneys. Although you won't experience generalized tissue swelling, it can contribute to the thickening of your heart and blood vessels.

If you have aldosteronism, your high blood pressure may be resistant to ordinary drug treatment. A low level of potassium in your blood also is a clue. Diagnostic steps include endocrine, urine and genetic tests, and CT or MRI examinations. Treatment may include drugs to block the action of aldosterone and surgery to remove a tumor.

Preeclampsia. Sometime after the 20th week of pregnancy, about 6 percent to 8 percent of pregnant women develop a condition called preeclampsia (pre-e-KLAMP-see-uh). It's characterized by a significant increase in blood pressure and excess protein in urine. Untreated, it can lead to serious, even deadly, complications for the mother and child. That's why blood pressure checks and urinalysis are routinely performed, particularly after midpregnancy.

After the baby is born, blood pressure usually returns to normal within several days to several weeks. Preeclampsia may recur during a subsequent pregnancy or it may indicate the possible development of future nonpregnancy hypertension. Preeclampsia is also discussed on pages 231-233.

Illicit drug use. Street drugs, such as cocaine and amphetamines, can lead to high blood pressure by narrowing certain arteries, increasing your heart rate or damaging your heart muscle.

Medications. Several types of drugs can increase blood pressure in some people. Over-the-counter (OTC) medications that may have this effect include:
- Cold remedies
- Nasal decongestants, including sprays
- Appetite suppressants
- Nonsteroidal anti-inflammatory drugs (NSAIDs) such as ibuprofen (Advil, Motrin) and naproxen sodium (Aleve)

Prescription medications that can affect blood pressure include:

- Steroids (prednisolone, methylprednisolone)
- Antidepressants (bupropion, desipramine, phenelzine, venlafaxine, others)
- Immunosuppressants (cyclosporine, tacrolimus, others)
- COX-2 inhibitors (celecoxib)
- Others (epoetin alfa, methylphenidate, sibutramine, yohimbine)

Most birth control pills can increase blood pressure, but the effect may be less pronounced in pills containing lower levels of estrogen. Drospirenone, a component of a contraceptive pill (Yasmin), can cause the body to retain potassium and interfere with certain medications for high blood pressure.

Sibutramine (Meridia), a prescription drug used for obesity, raises blood pressure substantially in some people.

Herbal supplements. Certain products associated with alternative and complementary medicine can increase blood pressure or interfere with the effectiveness of blood pressure medications. These include bitter orange, ginseng, licorice and St. John's wort.

The supplement ephedra (ma-huang) contains ephedrine, a chemical stimulant that has been linked to high blood pressure as well as other serious health problems. Herbal products containing ephedra have been marketed in the United States to promote weight loss and increase energy. In December 2003, the Food and Drug Administration banned ephedra from the marketplace because of health concerns.

It's always important to inform your doctor of all medications you're taking — prescription drugs, nonprescription drugs and herbal products. This is especially important if you're taking medication for high blood pressure.

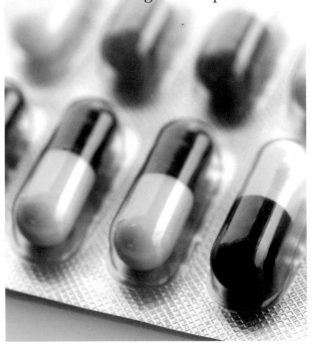

Identifying secondary high blood pressure

Similar to essential high blood pressure, you may not know you have secondary high blood pressure until your doctor has examined you and confirms it. Generally, with the secondary form, symptoms associated with the underlying condition may be the reasons that brought you to the doctor.

If it's discovered that you have high blood pressure, your doctor will want to know details of your medical history as well as of your family history. He or she likely will look for evidence of heart attack, heart disease, hardening of the arteries, weight change, leg pain during exercise, weakness and fatigue. The doctor will also check for signs and symptoms of conditions that can cause secondary high blood pressure.

Preventive action

High blood pressure is often preventable. You can help reduce your blood pressure and the risk of other cardiovascular diseases by eliminating or changing the risk factors that you can control. They include:

- Losing weight, if you're overweight
- Eating a healthy diet
- Becoming more physically active
- Stopping tobacco use
- Limiting alcohol

A healthier diet emphasizes lower fat and sodium intake, more vegetables, fruits and fiber, and reduced calories. Plan to be physically active for 30 to 60 minutes on most days of the week.

For many years, as long as your blood pressure was below the cutoff for being high, it was still considered to be at an acceptable level. That's no longer true. Doctors now know that prehypertension often develops into high blood pressure and increases your risk of cardiovascular disease.

Prehypertension refers to persistent systolic readings between 120 and 139 millimeters of mercury (mm Hg), diastolic readings between 80 and 89 mm Hg, or both. If your blood pressure is within these ranges, taking preventive measures is particularly important.

People with diabetes, heart disease or kidney disease should aim for a blood pressure of less than 130/80 mm Hg. In more severe cases of kidney disease and heart failure, a lower goal of 120/80 mm Hg may be recommended. In addition to lifestyle changes to lower blood pressure, these individuals may often require medications.

Weight and blood pressure

Changes in weight and blood pressure often go hand in hand. When your weight increases, your blood pressure often does, too. If you're overweight, your risk of developing high blood pressure is two to six times greater than if your weight is healthy.

Just as your blood pressure goes up when you gain weight, it usually goes down when you lose weight. Losing as little as 10 pounds can improve your blood pressure. If you're overweight, reducing your weight by 10 percent is a good goal to aim for. Weight loss can also improve your cholesterol levels and reduce your risk of heart attack, stroke, diabetes and arthritis.

What's the link between body weight and blood pressure? As you put on weight, you gain mostly fatty tissue, and this tissue relies on the nutrients in your blood to survive. As the demand for nutrients increases, the amount of circulating blood increases. More blood traveling through your arteries means greater pressure on your artery walls.

Another reason why blood pressure often increases when you're overweight is that additional weight typically raises your insulin level. More insulin is associated with the retention of sodium and water, which raises blood volume. In addition, excess body weight can increase your heart rate and reduce the capacity of your blood vessels to transport blood. Both factors can raise blood pressure.

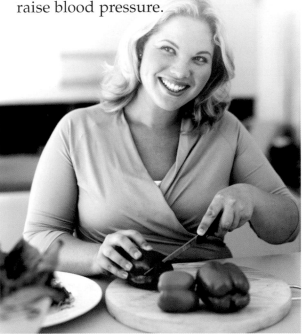

Recently, several naturally occurring chemicals have been identified that influence appetite, weight and blood pressure. For example, the hormone ghrelin helps trigger the urge to eat and the hormone leptin plays a role in suppressing the urge. Both hormones are under study.

What's become apparent is that interactions among these various chemicals are exceedingly complex, and there appears to be no direct relationship between hormone levels and weight control that can be used to regulate blood pressure.

Nevertheless, as the U.S. population has gotten heavier over the last few decades, weight control has become a major challenge in preventing high blood pressure.

Finding your healthy weight
The question you may be asking is, "How do I know what my healthy weight is supposed to be?" Technically, a healthy weight means you have the right amount of body fat in relation to your overall body mass. More than that, a healthy weight reduces your health risks, gives you energy, helps prevent premature aging and improves your quality of life.

The National Institutes of Health has adopted a threefold approach to determining a healthy weight. This approach is based on the following key components:
- Body mass index
- Waist circumference
- Medical history

The do-it-yourself evaluations that follow can help you determine whether your weight is healthy or whether you could benefit from losing a few more pounds. Doing so can help you control your blood pressure and also lessen your risks of other health problems.

Body mass index. Body mass index (BMI) is a standard formula that factors in your weight and your height in determining whether you have a healthy or unhealthy percentage of body fat. Except in very muscular people such as athletes, this measurement correlates well with total body fat.

To determine your BMI, locate your height on the chart on page 57 and follow it across until you reach the weight nearest yours. Look for the number at the top of the column for your BMI rating. If your weight is less than the weight nearest yours, your BMI may be slightly less. If your weight is greater

Body mass index (BMI)

You can determine your body mass index (BMI) by finding your height and weight on this chart. A BMI of 18.5 to 24.9 is considered the healthiest. People with a BMI under 18.5 are considered underweight. People with a BMI between 25 and 29.9 are considered overweight. People with a BMI of 30 or greater are considered obese.

	Healthy		Overweight					Obese				
BMI	**19**	**24**	**25**	**26**	**27**	**28**	**29**	**30**	**35**	**40**	**45**	**50**
Height							**Weight in pounds**					
4'10"	91	115	119	124	129	134	138	143	167	191	215	239
4'11"	94	119	124	128	133	138	143	148	173	198	222	247
5'0"	97	123	128	133	138	143	148	153	179	204	230	255
5'1"	100	127	132	137	143	148	153	158	185	211	238	264
5'2"	104	131	136	142	147	153	158	164	191	218	246	273
5'3"	107	135	141	146	152	158	163	169	197	225	254	282
5'4"	110	140	145	151	157	163	169	174	204	232	262	291
5'5"	114	144	150	156	162	168	174	180	210	240	270	300
5'6"	118	148	155	161	167	173	179	186	216	247	278	309
5'7"	121	153	159	166	172	178	185	191	223	255	287	319
5'8"	125	158	164	171	177	184	190	197	230	262	295	328
5'9"	128	162	169	176	182	189	196	203	236	270	304	338
5'10"	132	167	174	181	188	195	202	209	243	278	313	348
5'11"	136	172	179	186	193	200	208	215	250	286	322	358
6'0"	140	177	184	191	199	206	213	221	258	294	331	368
6'1"	144	182	189	197	204	212	219	227	265	302	340	378
6'2"	148	186	194	202	210	218	225	233	272	311	350	389
6'3"	152	192	200	208	216	224	232	240	279	319	359	399
6'4"	156	197	205	213	221	230	238	246	287	328	369	410

Note: Asians with a BMI of 23 or higher may have an increased risk of health problems. Source: National Institutes of Health, 1998

You can calculate your exact BMI by using this formula:

$$\left(\frac{\text{Weight in pounds}}{(\text{Height in inches}) \times (\text{Height in inches})} \right) \times 703 = \text{BMI}$$

For example, if you weigh 165 pounds and you're 5 feet 10 inches tall, your BMI is 23.7.

$$\left(\frac{165 \text{ pounds}}{(70 \text{ inches}) \times (70 \text{ inches})} \right) \times 703 = 23.7$$

than the weight nearest yours, your BMI may be slightly greater.

A BMI of 18.5 to 24.9 is considered healthy. A BMI of 25 to 29.9 signifies overweight, and a BMI of 30 or more indicates obesity. You're at increased risk of developing a weight-related disease, such as high blood pressure, if your BMI is 25 or greater. Asians with a BMI of 23 or greater may have an increased risk of health problems.

Waist circumference. This measurement — used in combination with your BMI — is also important in evaluating a healthy weight. It indicates where most of your fat is located.

Fat distribution can be described in terms of an apple shape or pear shape. If you carry most of your fat around your waist or upper body, you're referred to as apple shaped. If you carry most of your fat around your hips and thighs or lower body, you're referred to as pear shaped.

When it comes to your health, it's better to have a pear shape than an apple shape. If you have an apple shape, you carry fat around your abdominal organs, which increases your risk of high blood pressure, diabetes, abnor-

mal cholesterol levels, metabolic syndrome, coronary artery disease, stroke and certain types of cancer. If you have a pear shape, your risks of these conditions aren't as high.

To determine whether you have too much weight around your abdomen, measure your waist circumference. Find the highest point on each of your hipbones and measure across your abdomen just above those highest points. A measurement of more than 40 inches (102 centimeters or cm) in men and 35 inches (88 cm) in women signifies increased health risks, especially if your BMI is 25 or more.

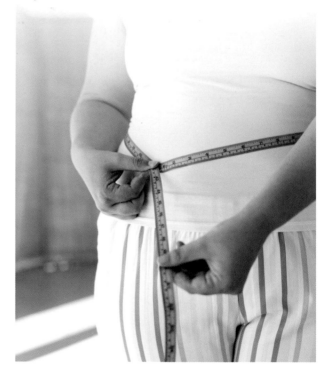

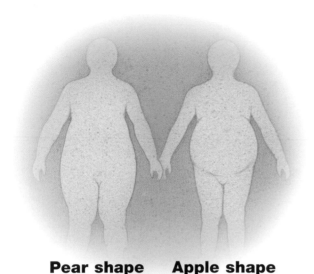

Pear shape   Apple shape

Fat distribution in your body

For Asians, the cutoff is slightly lower. Asian men should keep waist circumferences below 36 inches (90 cm) and Asian women below 32 inches (80 cm).

Although these cutoffs are useful guides, there's nothing magical about them. It's enough to know that the bigger your waistline, the greater your health risks.

Medical history. Numbers alone aren't enough. An evaluation of your medical history, as well as that of your family's history, is important for determining whether your weight is healthy.

Consider the following questions:
- Do you have a condition such as high blood pressure, type 2 diabetes or arthritis that would improve if you lost weight?
- Do you have a family history of a weight-related illness, such as high blood pressure, type 2 diabetes, high cholesterol, high triglycerides or sleep apnea?
- Have you gained considerable weight since high school? Even people with normal BMIs may be at increased risk of certain diseases if they've gained more than 10 pounds since young adulthood.
- Do you live with significant stress, smoke cigarettes, or have more than two alcoholic drinks a day if you're a man and more than one drink a day if you're a woman?

You can think of the BMI and waist measurement as snapshots of your current health status. Your medical history helps provide a more complete picture by revealing more about your risk of being overweight or developing weight-related diseases.

Adding up the results. If your BMI indicates you're not overweight and you're not carrying too much weight around your abdomen, there's proba-

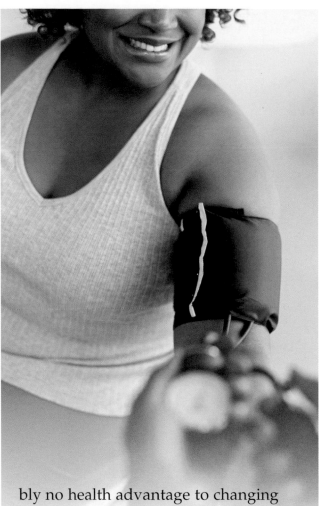

If your BMI is 30 or more, losing some weight will likely improve your health and reduce your risk of developing a weight-related illness.

Keys to successful weight loss

Despite the statistics you may have heard about how few people are able to lose weight, plenty of people do succeed. You can be one of them. Just because the task seems daunting doesn't mean that you shouldn't try. With a little knowledge, a positive attitude and a good plan, you can do it.

Here are guidelines that may help you lose weight safely and keep the pounds off permanently:

Make a commitment. Losing weight requires your full-time commitment. Don't dwell on what you're having to give up in order to lose weight. Concentrate instead on what you'll be gaining, including improved health and lower blood pressure.

Choose the right time. Timing is critical. If you're distracted or experiencing a difficult phase in your life, you may be less able to follow through on good intentions. It might be wise to postpone — but not cancel — weight loss as you resolve these problems.

bly no health advantage to changing your weight. You can consider your weight to be healthy.

If your BMI is between 25 and 29.9, you may benefit from losing a few more pounds, particularly if your waist circumference exceeds healthy guidelines or you answered yes to at least one of the medical history questions. Discuss options with your doctor at your next checkup.

Set realistic goals. Healthy weight loss is slow and steady. It involves losing no more that 1 to 2 pounds a week.

Learn new behaviors. Chances are that you've learned many eating habits in response to factors other than your empty stomach — social and emotional factors often come into play. The good news is that learned behaviors can also be unlearned over time.

But discarding a behavior or adopting a new one can take anywhere from three to 30 tries before you're successful. There's no magic formula that everyone can follow. You'll need to discover what's most effective for you.

Change gradually. The first rule of change is to not change too quickly — it's not a race. You're trying to develop a whole new lifestyle. This doesn't happen overnight.

Don't starve yourself. Extremely low-calorie diets and special food combinations aren't the answer to long-term weight control. Eating fewer than 1,200 calories makes it difficult for your body to get adequate amounts of nutrients. It also promotes temporary loss of fluids and of healthy muscle rather than the permanent loss of fat.

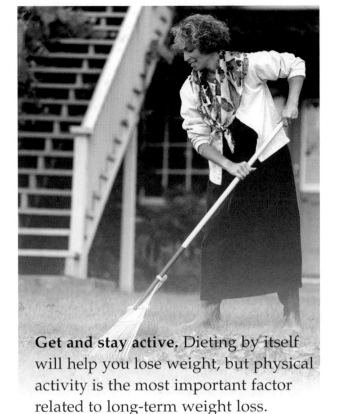

Get and stay active. Dieting by itself will help you lose weight, but physical activity is the most important factor related to long-term weight loss. Exercise promotes loss of body fat and development of muscle, making it easier to maintain weight loss.

Maintain your progress. Don't let minor setbacks weaken your resolve to lose weight. There will be days when you eat more than you'd planned or move less than you'd intended. It's inevitable that you'll occasionally lapse. It's important not to use a lapse as an excuse to give up. When it happens, rethink what you can do to put the healthy behavior back in your daily routine and stick with your plan.

Why act now?

You may wonder why it's so important to take steps to prevent high blood pressure. Why not simply wait for the condition to develop and then treat it, possibly with a little better diet and a little more activity?

In fact, there are many reasons why it's better to act now instead of waiting for later. Generally, the younger you are when you try to change your lifestyle, the better your chances are of succeeding at it. The longer you're able to maintain a healthy weight, the lower your risk of weight-related diseases.

Even with the successful treatment of blood pressure, changes to your heart and arteries may not reverse completely back to normal. It's better to prevent the damage from ever happening.

Wrap-up

Key points to remember:
- There are two forms of high blood pressure — essential and secondary. The cause of essential high blood pressure isn't known. Secondary high blood pressure results from an underlying illness or condition.
- Certain genetic or lifestyle factors place you at increased risk of developing high blood pressure. Generally, the more of these factors you have, the greater your risk.
- You may be able to prevent high blood pressure by eliminating or reducing certain risk factors that you can change.
- If you have prehypertension, reducing it to a normal level can help keep you from developing high blood pressure and cardiovascular disease as well as other diseases.

Chapter 3

Diagnosing high blood pressure

Unlike many other chronic health conditions, high blood pressure rarely produces signs and symptoms to warn you that something is wrong. Most people who have high blood pressure, even when the condition has been long term and uncontrolled, will look and feel just fine.

It's during routine medical examinations that most people learn that their blood pressure is too high. That's why it's important to have your blood pressure checked at least every two years. Otherwise, vital organs such as your heart and kidneys could be damaged without you even being aware of it.

Fortunately, diagnosing high blood pressure is a relatively straightforward process. It generally involves several measurements taken at doctor visits over a period of several weeks or months. This process confirms whether an initial high reading was simply a temporary fluctuation that returns to normal or represents what has become your regular level.

As part of the diagnostic process, your doctor likely will ask you questions about your health and your family's health, do a physical examination, and have you undergo routine tests. These steps are taken to determine whether any organs have been damaged by the high pressure levels. They may also prevent additional health problems from developing. Results from the examination and lab tests are also important in deciding how best to treat your condition. (See "Key questions to answer" on page 69.)

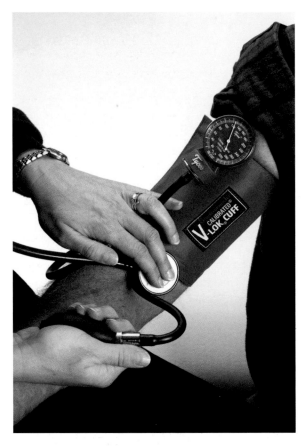

Sphygmomanometer

During a blood pressure reading, a doctor or nurse listens for sounds indicating your systolic and diastolic pressures.

Two methods for reducing and controlling high blood pressure are lifestyle changes and medication. Whether you'll need medication depends on your blood pressure, your risk of other health problems and whether any organ damage has occurred.

Taking a blood pressure reading

Measuring blood pressure is a simple procedure that you can learn to do. Here's how a reading is taken:

A sphygmomanometer (sfig-mo-muh-NOM-uh-tur) is the device that measures blood pressure. You're probably familiar with it from routine medical visits. The device includes an inflatable arm cuff with an attached air pump and a column of mercury or a standardized pressure gauge.

For a blood pressure measurement, the cuff is wrapped around your upper arm. Air is then pumped into the cuff by squeezing the bulb on the air pump. The cuff is inflated until the pressure inside it reaches a high level — well above the pressure that's required to

False readings

Sometimes, blood pressure measurements can produce false readings that are too high. This happens most often among older adults with damaged arteries that have become very stiff — and it's different from what's known as white-coat hypertension (see sidebar on page 68). Although many people with stiff arteries have high blood pressure, it may not be as high as the measurements indicate.

The false readings occur because rigid arteries are difficult to collapse. When a blood pressure measurement is taken, the cuff may not be able to collapse the brachial artery until the cuff has been inflated to extremely high pressure. And when pressure in the cuff is released, stiffness causes the artery to open faster than it normally should, which gives an incorrect reading.

Your doctor often can tell whether you have this condition, called pseudohypertension, by feeling your forearm. Normally, when a blood pressure cuff collapses your brachial artery, the doctor is unable to feel the arteries in your forearm below the cuff.

Stiff arteries in the forearm, however, remain open and can be felt even when no blood is flowing through them. People with this condition may find that electronic devices also fail to give accurate readings.

To get an accurate measurement with pseudohypertension, you may need to have the pressure in your arteries measured by inserting a needle into the brachial artery or into the radial artery in your forearm.

push blood through your blood vessels. This causes the main artery in your arm (brachial artery) to collapse, cutting off blood flow to the rest of your arm. When the artery collapses, no sounds are heard through a stethoscope that's placed over the artery, just below the cuff.

Air is then slowly released from the cuff, gradually reducing pressure on your collapsed artery. As soon as pressure in the cuff equals your systolic pressure, blood begins to flow through your artery once again. This causes thumping sounds that can be heard through the stethoscope.

The number on the mercury column or pressure gauge at the moment that a doctor, nurse or technician hears the return of blood flow to your arm indicates your systolic pressure (written as the upper number).

As air continues to be released from the cuff, pressure on the brachial artery continues to drop. When the artery is fully open again, the thumping sounds become inaudible. The reading on the mercury column or pressure gauge at the moment the sounds disappear indicates your diastolic pressure (written as the lower number).

Electronic sphygmomanometers include a fully automatic monitor. The electronic units inflate and deflate the cuff, detect your systolic and diastolic pressures by sensing vibrations in the artery, and then display your measurements on a digital screen.

To produce accurate readings, the inflatable part of the cuff needs to cover at least three-quarters of your upper arm. If you will be measuring your blood pressure, see Chapter 4 for instructions and advice on the devices. Also ask your doctor for help.

Making certain

A blood pressure reading of 140/90 millimeters of mercury (mm Hg) is considered high. But a single reading of 140/90 mm Hg or higher usually isn't enough for a diagnosis of high blood pressure. Your blood pressure varies throughout the day, and it's best to obtain multiple readings under circumstances that are similar. Only if the reading is extremely high — a systolic pressure of 180 mm Hg or higher or a diastolic pressure of 110 mm Hg or higher — is a diagnosis made based on a single measurement.

Generally, a diagnosis of high blood pressure is made after at least two visits to your doctor. Your blood pressure is measured two or more times at each visit, for a total of at least four measurements. If the average of the four measurements shows your blood pressure to be 140/90 mm Hg or higher, then you have high blood pressure.

If you're older than 65 years, the doctor may require even more measurements because, as you get older, there are many more reasons why your blood pressure readings may vary, including stiffened arteries (see page 65).

To ensure an accurate reading, don't smoke, eat a big meal, or drink caffeine or alcohol for at least 30 minutes before taking your blood pressure. And make sure your bladder is empty. All of these factors can temporarily increase blood pressure for a period of time.

Also give yourself plenty of time to make your appointment. Rushing around can cause stress, which can temporarily increase blood pressure. Before you have your blood pressure measured, sit quietly for two to five minutes with your back supported and both feet flat on the floor.

Why do I need to return for more blood pressure readings after my first visit?

Let's say that at a routine medical exam, your blood pressure reading was above 140/90 mm Hg. Unless your blood pressure was extremely high (180/110 mm Hg or higher), you'll need to return for additional checks. That's because many factors can affect your blood pressure, and measurements vary widely throughout the day and from day to day. At least two measurements are taken at each subsequent visit, generally under identical circumstances. A fair gauge of your regular blood pressure is the average of these measurements from all your visits.

White-coat hypertension and masked hypertension

Some people become anxious whenever their blood pressure is measured at the doctor's office. They may have normal blood pressure at other times and at other places, but whenever it's measured in a medical setting, it's always going to be high. This condition, called white-coat hypertension, occurs in around 10 percent to 30 percent of people with high blood pressure.

For other people, the opposite holds true. Their blood pressure consistently measures higher when they're at home or at work than it does when they visit the doctor's office. This condition is called masked hypertension. It may occur for several reasons. For example, the calm, quiet environment at the doctor's office may be less stressful than the other environments they live in.

If your doctor suspects your high blood pressure is white-coat hypertension, you may need to keep track of your blood pressure away from a medical setting. For both white-coat and masked hypertension, your doctor may recommend that you wear a portable device (ambulatory monitor) that measures your blood pressure periodically over a 24-hour period while you go about your regular activities. For either condition, this method can generally provide you with a more realistic and accurate assessment of your blood pressure.

Automated machines in stores and shopping malls that measure blood pressure aren't recommended for this purpose. These machines are not sufficiently accurate, and they're often equipped with cuffs that don't fit properly. Furthermore, the settings where these machines are located — which can have a huge impact on blood pressure readings — aren't controlled and, in fact, can even be chaotic.

Conventional medical thought has been that these forms of hypertension are harmless phenomena not requiring treatment. In fact, many people with these conditions will develop true hypertension over time. A recent study suggests that masked hypertension may put you at higher risk of stroke and death from cardiovascular disease. Both conditions should be carefully monitored and treated. Your doctor may recommend adjustments to your lifestyle and blood pressure medications.

When having your blood pressure taken, don't talk. Talking can elevate blood pressure as well as make it harder for the person taking the measurement to hear the sound of your heartbeat. Some offices now have an automatic device that takes readings every few minutes while you're alone, quiet and seated properly.

Key questions to answer

Between the time you first learn that you may have high blood pressure and the time of an actual diagnosis, your doctor may want to get your medical history, perform a complete physical examination and have you undergo several lab tests.

These three components can provide answers to important diagnostic questions, such as:

- Has your high blood pressure damaged any organs?
- Is your high blood pressure essential (primary) or secondary? Although secondary high blood pressure is uncommon, it's important that each person with high

blood pressure be considered for secondary causes. Some of these conditions are treatable, allowing you to reduce blood pressure.

- Do you have other risk factors that increase your chances of having a heart attack or stroke, such as tobacco use, too much weight, an inactive lifestyle, high blood cholesterol or diabetes?

If it's unclear whether you have high blood pressure or prehypertension, these evaluations can help confirm the diagnosis and guide treatment decisions for the condition.

Medical history

Your medical history may point to a particular factor or event that has triggered the increase in blood pressure. This history can also help the doctor assess your risk of other health conditions. During an evaluation, you may be asked questions regarding:

- Previous blood pressure readings
- Personal history of heart disease, kidney disease, high cholesterol, diabetes and sleep apnea (for example, snoring, restless sleep or daytime sleepiness)

Round-the-clock reading

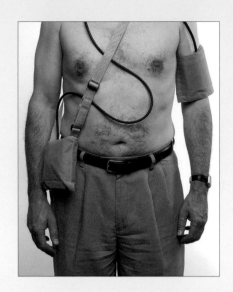

High blood pressure can, at times, be difficult to diagnose. If your doctor is uncertain whether or not you have high blood pressure and if so, how severe it is, you may need to wear a special device known as an ambulatory monitor.

This device is a portable blood pressure monitor that you can wear for a day. It includes an inflatable cuff that fits around your arm and a small monitoring unit that hangs at your waist using a strap over your shoulder. A thin tube connecting the monitor to the cuff may be secured to your skin with tape to prevent it from twisting or disconnecting.

The monitor is programmed to take your blood pressure about every 10 to 30 minutes over a period of six to 24 hours. The device is fully automatic. At selected times, it pumps up the blood pressure cuff, deflates it, takes a reading and stores the information in its memory.

You may be a candidate for ambulatory monitoring if you have white-coat hypertension — your blood pressure readings are higher than normal only at medical checkups — or masked hypertension — you show complications of high blood pressure but have normal blood pressure readings at medical checkups. Ambulatory monitoring can also be helpful if your blood pressure fluctuates widely or if you're not responding to treatment with blood pressure medications.

While wearing the monitor, keep a journal that lists your daily activities and the times you did them, the times you took medications, and any periods of stress, strong emotions or pain. By comparing the journal entries with your blood pressure readings from the ambulatory monitor, your doctor may note where certain events or lifestyle factors are linked to changes in your blood pressure.

- Family history of high blood pressure, heart attack, stroke, kidney disease, diabetes, high cholesterol or early (premature) death
- Signs and symptoms that may suggest secondary high blood pressure, such as flushing spells, rapid heart rate, intolerance of heat or unexplained weight loss

You may also be asked questions about your behaviors and habits related to:
- Alcohol use
- Diet and use of salt (sodium)
- Tobacco use
- Medications you're currently taking and previous use of high blood pressure drugs
- Changes in weight
- Activity level

Inform your doctor of all medications you take — both prescription and over-the-counter (OTC), as well as illicit drugs and herbal and nutritional supplements. Note any drugs that you've had adverse reaction or intolerance to.

Compile a list of these medications, including drug names and dosages. If you don't have a list, bring the original containers with you to your next doctor visit. For more information about medications, see Step 5 in this book.

Various prescription and OTC drugs can increase your blood pressure, as well as street drugs such as cocaine. Because the health effects of many supplements haven't been fully studied, it's important to tell your doctor if you're taking one of these products, in case it affects blood pressure.

Keeping your doctor aware of all of the drugs you take can also prevent dangerous drug interactions. Some blood pressure medications don't react well with other drugs.

Keep in mind that blood pressure normally rises and falls over a 24-hour period. Diet, activities, emotions and other factors also affect blood pressure. These variations must be taken into account as you and your doctor consider your use of medications.

Physical examination

Your doctor will examine your body closely for signs of organ damage. He or she will also check for abnormalities that signal a possible cause for the blood pressure increase.

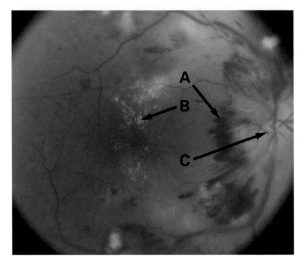 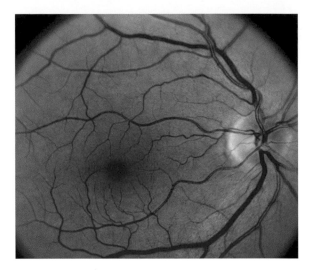

Damage to the retina

Shown on the left, blood vessels in your retina may rupture due to high blood pressure, causing bleeding (hemorrhaging, see A) and a buildup of waste deposits (exudates, see B). Tissue swelling due to a combination of leakage and inflammation may include the optic nerve (papilledema, see C). The image of a healthy retina is shown on the right.

Physical conditions that your doctor may consider when checking for signs of organ damage include:

Narrowed or leaky blood vessels in your eyes. Damage to the blood vessels in your eyes is a strong indicator that blood vessels elsewhere in your body have been damaged by high pressure. This may also indicate an increased risk of cardiovascular disease.

Heart abnormalities. A fast heart rate, a heart that's enlarged in size, an abnormal rhythm of your heartbeat, or a click or murmur in the sounds of the heart can signal possible heart disease.

Turbulent blood flow. When a blood vessel narrows, it can cause turbulent blood flow. The turbulent flow, called a bruit (BRU-we), most often occurs in the carotid arteries in your neck and the major arteries in your abdomen.

Decreased blood pressure when you stand. A side effect of some blood pressure medications is fainting or dizziness when you stand up (postural hypotension). Such dizziness is also a complication of diabetes. The problem is common in older adults particularly after meals, whether or not they have diabetes. For more information, see "When your blood pressure drops too low" on page 30.

Aortic aneurysm. An aneurysm can form at a weak spot in the wall of the aorta. A bulge may be felt during an examination of your abdomen. A stethoscope also may pick up the sound of blood pulsing through the weakened blood vessel.

Weakened pulse. A weak pulse in your groin, lower legs and ankles can signal artery damage.

Reduced blood pressure in your ankles. This can result from narrowed or diseased blood vessels in your legs.

Swelling. Accumulation of fluid in your lower legs and ankles is a common sign of heart or kidney failure.

Enlarged kidneys or thyroid gland. If either of these organs becomes enlarged, it may indicate that you have secondary high blood pressure resulting from another condition.

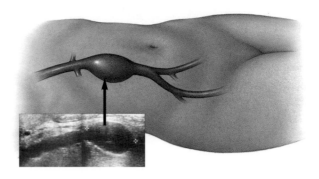

Aortic aneurysm

An aortic aneurysm is a bulging section in the wall of the aorta (see arrow) that may rupture or be the location of blood clot formation. Aneurysms can be detected with an ultrasound image (see inset).

Routine tests

The following tests are commonly included in a routine evaluation for high blood pressure:

Weight. Being overweight or obese may play a role in raising your blood pressure. Your weight usually is taken as part of a general office visit.

Your doctor may calculate your body mass index (BMI) to determine whether you have an unhealthy percentage of body fat (see pages 56-58). In addition, your doctor may also measure your waist to determine whether you're carrying too much weight around your abdomen (see pages 58-59).

Urinalysis. The presence of protein or red blood cells in your urine can indicate kidney damage. A form of protein in your urine, called microalbuminuria (mi-kro-al-bu-min-U-ree-uh), can also signal early-stage kidney disease — a risk factor for future cardiovascular disease. In addition, your urine may be tested for the presence of sugar (glucose) resulting from diabetes. Diabetes can make high blood pressure more difficult to control.

Blood chemistry. The levels of sodium and potassium in your blood are measured. Your blood may also be tested for levels of the compound creatinine (kre-AT-ih-nin), which can indicate damage to your kidneys.

Other common blood tests include measurements of cholesterol-containing blood fats (lipid profile). The higher your total blood cholesterol level and the lower your high-density lipoprotein (HDL, or "good") cholesterol level, the greater your risk of cardiovascular disease and metabolic syndrome. The level of glucose (sugar) in your blood may also be measured to check for diabetes.

Complete blood cell count. This test reveals abnormal white and red blood cell counts. Its purpose is to ensure that you don't have certain health conditions you may not be aware of, such as a low red blood cell count, called anemia (uh-NE-me-uh).

Electrocardiography. Your heart's electrical activity is monitored to check for rhythm abnormalities or indications of damage, including an enlarged heart or inadequate blood supply.

The changes in your heart's electrical activity is recorded on an electrocardiogram (ECG), which can also indicate high or low levels of potassium.

Additional tests

If your physical examination and laboratory findings are normal, you probably won't have to undergo additional testing. However, further tests may be necessary if you have:
- Sudden onset of high blood pressure or a sharp increase in your normal blood pressure
- Very high blood pressure (180 or higher/110 or higher mm Hg)

- Low blood potassium level
- Sound of turbulent blood flow (bruit) heard over an artery
- Evidence of kidney problems
- Evidence of heart problems
- Indications of an abdominal aortic aneurysm

If you have narrowed arteries that are interrupting blood flow, imaging tests can identify the location and severity of the problem:

Angiography. This procedure injects a dye into the blood vessels of your body that's highly visible to an X-ray machine. The X-ray machine rapidly takes a series of images (angiograms) that reveal many hidden or subtle features of your arteries.

Magnetic resonance angiography (MRA). Rather than using X-rays to produce an image, magnetic resonance imaging uses magnetic fields and radio waves. The device detects and stores small energy signals emitted by the atoms that make up body tissue. A computer program reconstructs images based on this information.

Ultrasonography. This procedure uses high-frequency sound waves to track the function of your circulatory system.

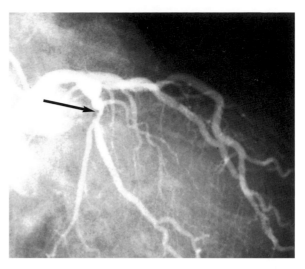

Coronary arteriogram

This angiogram shows partial blockage in a coronary artery (see arrow), which restricts blood flow to the heart muscle.

The waves bounce off internal structures and back to a transducer, which converts the reflected waves into a distinct image (see example on page 73).

If your doctor suspects that you may have a shrunken kidney, an abdominal aortic aneurysm or an adrenal gland tumor, additional tests may include:

Magnetic resonance imaging (MRI). This procedure is based on the same principles as the MRA, but provides detailed images of organs rather than blood vessels.

Computerized tomography (CT). The image produced in a CT scan is generated by an X-ray beam, but this technology provides much more information than an ordinary X-ray. That's because the doughnut-shaped machine contains a rotating scanner that emits a series of beams from all angles around your body. A computer gathers these X-ray signals and processes them into highly detailed, 3-D images of your internal organs.

Nuclear scanning. After radioactive material is injected into a vein, nuclear images are taken that show the material passing through a specific location or organ. Nuclear scans are used to monitor blood flow and to determine the size and function of organs.

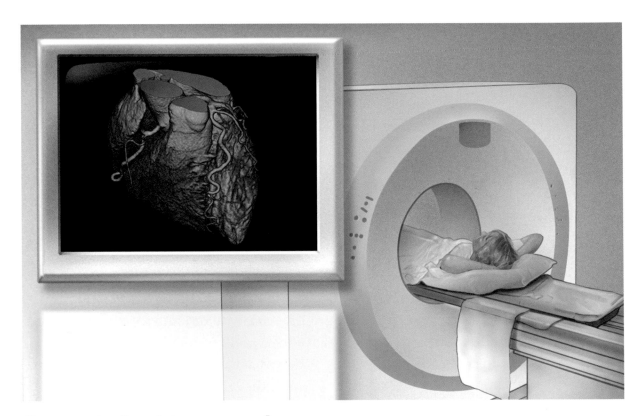

Computerized tomography

A computerized tomography scan involves taking multiple, highly specialized X-rays of an organ such as the heart. With the help of computer programs, highly detailed images of the heart and blood vessels can be created.

Deciding on a treatment plan

Treatment of high blood pressure should be tailored to your individual needs. That's why the type of treatment that works for someone else may not be the best fit for you. You and your doctor will need to consider your medical history, a current physical examination and the results of laboratory tests to determine the most effective, personalized plan.

There are two basic approaches to reducing high blood pressure — changing unhealthy aspects of your lifestyle and taking medications. Depending on your health and risk factors, recommended lifestyle changes may include losing weight, becoming more active, eating a healthier diet, reducing sodium, stopping smoking, limiting alcohol and controlling stress.

Several types of medications are used to control high blood pressure, and there are new developments on the horizon. Genetic research suggests that heredity may potentially be used to match individuals with certain medications to increase the efficacy of drugs.

These medications affect blood pressure in different ways. It's important not to share the drugs prescribed for you with anyone else. Their medication may not be the same type as yours.

Latest guidelines

The National Heart, Lung, and Blood Institute (NHLBI), a division of the National Institutes of Health, periodically issues a report called the Joint National Committee on Prevention, Detection, Evaluation, and Treatment of High Blood Pressure. The seventh report was issued in 2003 and is often referred to as JNC 7.

The report divides elevated blood pressure into three categories — prehypertension, stage 1 hypertension and stage 2 hypertension. JNC 7 also makes treatment recommendations for people in each category (see page 78).

The risk of cardiovascular disease, stroke and kidney disease is determined according to your blood pressure, the condition of your internal organs and the presence of other risk factors, combined with any cardiovascular damage. If you have prehypertension and can't lower your blood pressure, there's a good chance that a

Guidelines for treatment

Blood pressure level (mm Hg)	Treatment
Normal (119/79 or lower)	Pursue a healthy lifestyle
Prehypertension (120-139/or 80-89)	Adopt a healthy lifestyle
Stage 1 (140-159/or 90-99)	Lifestyle changes,* plus a medication
Stage 2 (≥160/or ≥100)	Lifestyle changes, plus more than one medication

*If you don't have risk factors, your doctor may first recommend a short trial of lifestyle changes alone without medication.

Major risk factors that can affect treatment

Tobacco use

Undesirable blood fat (lipid) levels

Physical inactivity

Obesity (BMI ≥30)

Diabetes

Impaired kidney function

Age (>55 for men, >65 for women)

Sex (male, or post-menopausal female)

Family history of cardiovascular disease (age <55 for men, age <65 for women)

Organ damage or disease that can affect treatment

Heart disease

Muscle thickening in main pumping chamber

Previous heart attack or chest pain (angina)

Prior bypass surgery or angioplasty

Heart failure

Stroke or transient ischemic attack (ministroke)

Chronic kidney disease

Peripheral artery damage

Retinal damage

Adapted from the National Institutes of Health. The Seventh Report of the Joint National Committee on Prevention, Detection, Evaluation, and Treatment of High Blood Pressure, 2003

Numbers on progress are mixed

Since 1972, when the NHLBI began an intensive education campaign, there generally has been steady improvement in awareness, treatment and control of high blood pressure. As a result, death and disability attributed to the disease have declined significantly. Death rates from stroke have dropped by nearly 70 percent, and deaths due to heart attack have declined by more than 60 percent.

During the early 1990s, those dramatic improvements slowed. The reasons for the slowdown are unclear. An increase in obesity and lack of exercise may be factors. In *Health, United States, 2002*, a report by the Surgeon General, it noted that three in five adults ages 20 to 74 were overweight, and that one in four Americans was considered to be obese. The report also noted that nearly 40 percent of Americans engage in no physical activity during leisure time.

Another factor may be complacency. Above-normal blood pressures too often may be overlooked — both by doctors and their patients — as being "almost" in control and therefore not of great concern.

Despite these findings, there is also good news. Data gathered in the National Health and Nutrition Examination Survey (NHANES) on people with high blood pressure, as well as data on patient care through managed care organizations and the Veterans Affairs showed improvement in blood pressure control rates. The control rate improved from 29 percent in 1999 to 2000 to 37 percent in 2003 to 2004. These improvements were particularly strong in adults over the age of 60.

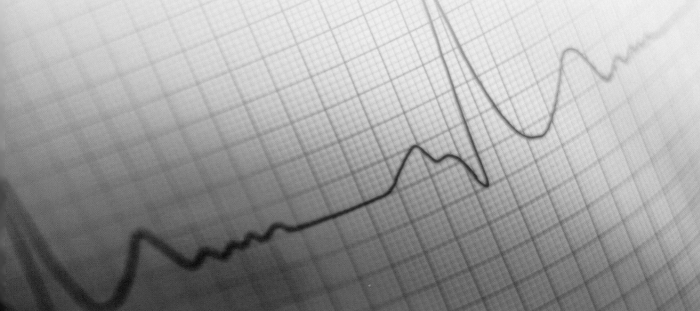

cardiovascular event will occur and you'll develop stage 1 hypertension.

Recent guidelines from institutions outside the United States — for example, European Society of Hypertension-European Society of Cardiology, World Health Organization-International Society of Hypertension, the British Hypertension Society and the Canadian Hypertension Society — take a similar approach. Recent studies have provided evidence supporting blood pressure goals even lower than those set by some of these organizations in certain circumstances.

The treatment of prehypertension and hypertension is based on a number of important factors. They include whether or not you have cardiovascular disease or have any risk factors for it. Also taken into account is your systolic and diastolic blood pressure.

While the treatment goal will always be the same — to lower your blood pressure — the number of risk factors you have will determine how aggressively your blood pressure is treated. Special attention will be given to addressing the reversible risk factors, such as tobacco use, high cholesterol levels and diabetes.

Prehypertension. If you have prehypertension, you're at increased risk of sustained hypertension and developing cardiovascular complications. You'll be encouraged to adopt lifestyle changes designed to reduce your blood pressure to a lower level (see sidebar on page 78.) If you have kidney disease, heart disease or diabetes, medication may also be required.

Stage 1 hypertension. If you're in the stage 1 level of hypertension, lifestyle changes are part of the first-line treatment. You'll likely also need a blood pressure lowering medication to bring your blood pressure under control. For most people with stage 1 hypertension, a thiazide diuretic may be one of the most effective options. Other choices include an angiotensin-converting enzyme (ACE) inhibitor, angiotensin II receptor blocker (ARB) or calcium channel blocker (CCB).

Stage 2 hypertension. Individuals in this category are at greatest risk of heart attack, stroke or other problems related to high blood pressure. A combination of two drugs along with changes in lifestyle are typically recommended. Medications may include a thiazide diuretic used with an ACE inhibitor, ARB, CCB or renin inhibitor.

Refining treatment goals

Your treatment plan for high blood pressure will include specific goals that take into account other factors in addition to your blood pressure level and unhealthy behaviors. For example, your doctor will also consider your overall health and the presence of other diseases and conditions.

If you have diabetes or kidney disease or have had heart disease, stroke or a transient ischemic attack, your target blood pressure may be set at less than 130/80 mm Hg to further reduce your risk of complications. (Note that the low end of the range for stage 1 high blood pressure is 140/90 mm Hg.) If you have severe kidney or heart disease, your doctor may advise a goal of less than 120/75 mm Hg.

Common misconception

Many people taking high blood pressure medication believe that it's not as important to make changes in their lifestyle simply because their medication is taking care of the problem. That's not true.

Sometimes, medication can reduce your blood pressure by only a certain amount. And that amount may not be enough to reach your blood pressure target level. However, succeeding with lifestyle changes in addition to taking medication often can help you reach the target pressure.

If you're able to reach a target blood pressure with medication, making lifestyle changes may help reduce the amount of medication you need. Less medication usually means less cost. If your medication causes bothersome side effects, cutting back on the dosage may reduce them. Some people who've significantly changed their lifestyle have been able to stop taking medication entirely.

Finally, lifestyle changes are important for all people with high blood pressure because they help reduce risk of stroke, heart attack, heart failure, kidney failure and dementia.

Achieving your target goals generally requires your full involvement. Meet with your doctor regularly to assess your progress and to adjust your treatment plan. Reaching your goal sooner results in less risk of cardiovascular events occurring, so don't wait for more than a few months for lifestyle changes or medications to work.

How do I manage the lifestyle changes?

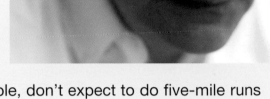

It can be overwhelming to try and adjust your diet, start exercising, lower stress, stop smoking and watch your alcohol intake all at once. Here are general rules that may guide your decisions and keep you on track:

First, keep your goals realistic. If you set your expectations too high or hold yourself to impossible goals, you're setting yourself up for failure. For example, don't expect to do five-mile runs as soon as you start jogging.

Second, don't try to change too quickly. This is not a race. You're trying to develop a new lifestyle, and ridding yourself of habits you've probably followed for many years. This doesn't happen overnight.

Third, it's important that you enjoy and find satisfaction in the changes you're making to your lifestyle. If you don't like what you're doing, it's unlikely you'll stay with the plan.

Fourth, it's inevitable that you'll have an occasional lapse, for example, when travel or work deadlines cause you to eat poorly and not exercise. When this happens, don't get discouraged and get back on your plan.

Fifth, stay focused on your health. Remind yourself that being healthy allows you to be energetic, strong, active and experience an optimum quality of life.

Being an active partner

You can live a long and healthy life with high blood pressure. But to do so, you need to recognize that high blood pressure is a serious condition that you can bring under control. If you're diagnosed with high blood pressure or considered to be at high risk of the condition, your doctor may ask you to make fundamental changes to your lifestyle. This makes you an active participant in your health care.

The chapters in Part 2 of this book describe five steps for controlling high blood pressure: Eating well, being more active, stopping smoking and limiting alcohol, reducing stress and getting the right medications. These steps can guide you in assuming day-to-day responsibilities for the treatment plan that your doctor sets up for you.

Recognize that it takes a team effort to treat high blood pressure. You can't do it alone, and you can't depend on your doctor to do it for you. Everyone working together and supporting you, including family and friends, can help you achieve your goals.

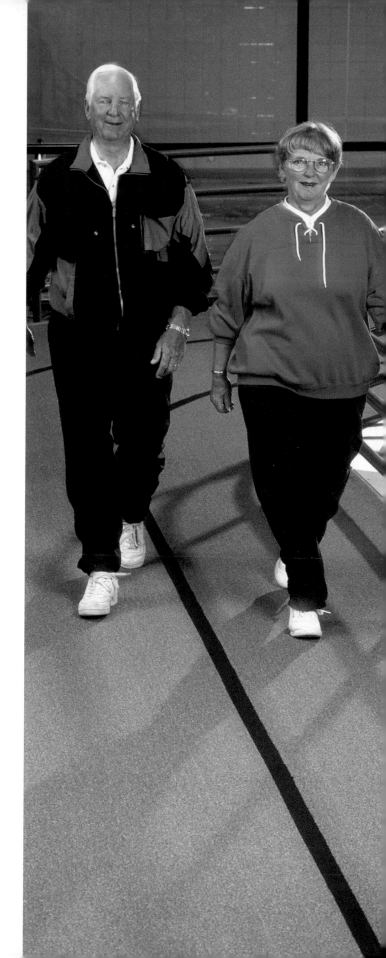

Wrap-up

Key points to remember:
- Many factors can influence a single blood pressure reading including diet, activity, fluid intake, stress level, posture and time of day.
- A high blood pressure diagnosis generally is made after multiple readings show persistently high systolic or diastolic pressure, or both.
- A medical history, physical examination and routine lab tests are typically part of the process to diagnose high blood pressure.
- Appropriate treatment of high blood pressure depends on blood pressure stage, organ damage, cardiovascular risk factors, and the presence of diabetes or other diseases.
- Even if you take medication, changes in your lifestyle are essential to controlling high blood pressure.

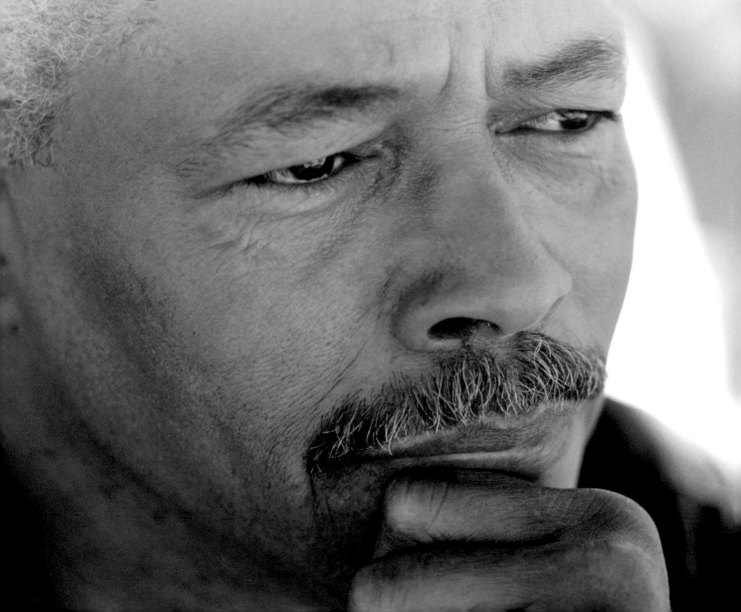

Part 2

Five steps to control high blood pressure

Step 1

Eat smart

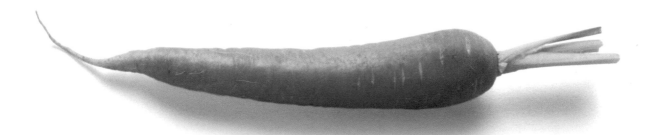

Of all the factors that influence blood pressure, your diet may be one that you can do the most about. You can't change your genes and you can't stop aging, but you can certainly decide what food to put on your plate.

By choosing healthier foods, you can lower your blood pressure and keep it under better control. Even modest changes can make a significant difference. A healthy diet, along with physical activity and other lifestyle changes, can lessen the chance that you'll need medication to treat high blood pressure. Or it may mean you'll take fewer medications or at a lower dose.

As the assessments in the introduction of this book suggest, the benefits of a healthy diet extend beyond blood pressure to heart health and overall good health — reducing your risk of stroke, heart attack, heart failure and kidney failure. Eating well can also help you lose weight or avoid gaining weight, important factors in managing your blood pressure.

Eating smart to manage high blood pressure involves more than just cutting down on your salt intake. For decades, public health officials told people with high blood pressure to limit sodium in their diet. This advice still holds, but it turns out that salt is just one part of the story. Recent studies have shown that other aspects of your diet, including your eating behaviors, can affect blood pressure. A comprehensive approach to food makes more sense than focusing solely on salt.

And eating smart doesn't mean counting calories and giving up the foods you like. You can enjoy a variety of foods that keep you healthy in the years ahead. Read on to learn more about what to eat more of, what to eat less of and how to incorporate good eating behaviors into your daily life.

Healthy-eating basics

Over the years, many studies have demonstrated the benefits of eating healthy. But exactly what is meant by a "healthy diet?" It's more than just calorie counting. Quite simply, a healthy diet is rich in fruits, vegetables, whole grains and low-fat or fat-free dairy products. By emphasizing these foods, such a diet limits fat, cholesterol and calories while providing plentiful amounts of nutrients and fiber.

One such approach is the DASH diet. Known officially as Dietary Approaches to Stop Hypertension (DASH), it provides a lifelong approach to healthy eating. The DASH diet stems from several key studies that compared various eating plans.

In the first study, people with or at risk of high blood pressure followed one of three diets — a "typical" American diet, the DASH diet, or a diet that promoted fruits and vegetables but didn't limit dairy products or fat. Participants who ate the DASH diet were able to reduce their blood pressure significantly — and within two weeks. African-American participants and those with high blood pressure experienced the most dramatic drops. The DASH diet also lowered levels of low-density lipoprotein (LDL or "bad") cholesterol.

The initial DASH diet included about 3,000 milligrams (mg) daily of sodium — less than what most Americans consume on a daily basis. A follow-up study, called DASH-Sodium, found that consuming less salt brought an even greater reduction in blood pressure. Participants who consumed no more than 1,500 mg of sodium a day experienced the greatest reductions in their blood pressure.

In the OmniHeart Trial, researchers modified the DASH diet by replacing some carbohydrates with either more protein or more unsaturated fat. Both diets lowered blood pressure further — and also improved triglyceride and cholesterol levels, possibly reducing the risk of coronary artery disease.

Other dietary options

Other eating plans share a similar premise as the DASH diet. One such plan is the Mayo Clinic Healthy Weight Pyramid, which is designed to help you achieve and maintain a healthy weight. Like the DASH diet, the Healthy Weight Pyramid promotes eating more whole grains, fruits and vegetables and fewer animal products, including meat, poultry and fish. The DASH plan differs in that it separates vegetable proteins from animal proteins, recommending four to five servings a week of nuts, seeds and legumes (vegetable protein sources).

A lower carb approach

The OmniHeart study showed that replacing some carbohydrates with either protein or monounsaturated fat lowers blood pressure even more than in the regular DASH diet. But increased protein intake doesn't translate into just eating more bacon and steak. About two-thirds of the added protein in the study came from plant sources, including legumes, grains, nuts and seeds. The diet higher in monounsaturated fat included more olive, canola and safflower oils, as well as nuts and seeds.

If you're interested in a lower carb approach, don't forget to pay attention to overall calories. Fats have more calories per serving than carbohydrates and proteins do. If you substitute fats for carbohydrates, make sure to adjust daily servings to meet your calorie goal.

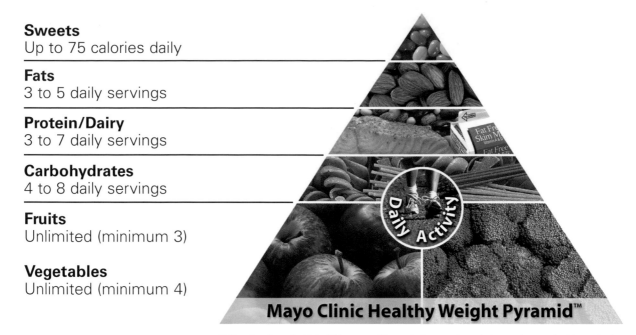

Sweets
Up to 75 calories daily

Fats
3 to 5 daily servings

Protein/Dairy
3 to 7 daily servings

Carbohydrates
4 to 8 daily servings

Fruits
Unlimited (minimum 3)

Vegetables
Unlimited (minimum 4)

Mayo Clinic Healthy Weight Pyramid™

© Mayo Foundation for Medical Education and Research. See your doctor before you begin any healthy weight plan.

Mayo Clinic Healthy Weight Pyramid

The DASH diet is similar in many respects to the Mayo Clinic Healthy Weight Pyramid — the principles of which can provide a healthy-eating plan for most Americans. Both dietary approaches emphasize greater consumption of fruits, vegetables and carbohydrate-containing whole grain products and less consumption of meat.

Another eating plan that can help control high blood pressure is known as the Mediterranean diet. Rooted in the traditional diets of countries such as Greece and Italy, the Mediterranean diet includes a generous amount of fruits, vegetables, olive oil, legumes, nuts, pasta, rice and bread. Moderate amounts of fish, dairy products, wine and beans are consumed, while red meat is eaten sparingly.

Compared with the DASH diet, the Mediterranean diet includes a greater amount of unsaturated fats, mainly from the use of olive oil, nuts and fish. Considered heart healthy, these fat sources do not raise blood cholesterol

Daily calorie goals

The number of calories that most adults should eat in a day ranges from 1,600 to 2,400 daily calories. A servings guide for the DASH diet is typically set at 2,100 daily calories. To lose weight, it's recommended that an average woman set her calorie goal at 1,200 calories, and an average man at 1,400 calories — if their weight is at or below 250 pounds. Consult your doctor or registered dietitian if you have questions about your calorie goal.

levels. Several studies showed that people who ate a Mediterranean-style diet lowered their blood pressure as much as did people who followed the regular DASH diet, but less than did people on the low-sodium DASH diet.

Discuss with a doctor or registered dietitian about which eating plan may suit your health and eating preferences best. For many people with high blood pressure, it makes sense to start with the DASH diet. A recent study found individuals with prehypertension and stage 1 hypertension who combined the DASH diet with comprehensive lifestyle changes that included weight loss, physical activity, and reduced sodium and alcohol intake were able to achieve better blood pressure control.

The DASH diet

The DASH eating plan focuses on foods rich in nutrients that can help lower blood pressure, including essential minerals such as potassium, calcium and magnesium.

In addition to plentiful amounts of fruits and vegetables, DASH includes whole grains, low-fat dairy products, poultry, fish and nuts. This diet follows heart-healthy guidelines by limiting saturated fat and cholesterol, as well as reducing intake of red meat, sweets and sugary beverages. The DASH-Sodium study demonstrated that the greatest reduction in blood pressure occurred by including lower sodium intake with a healthy diet.

The DASH eating plan

Food group	Daily servings	Serving sizes
Whole grains	6 to 8	½ cup (3 oz/90 g) cooked rice, pasta or cereal 1 oz (30 g) ready-to-eat (dry) cereal (serving size varies between ½ cup and 1-¼ cups, depending on cereal type) 1 slice bread ½ English muffin
Vegetables	4 to 5	1 cup (2 oz/60 g) raw leafy vegetables ½ cup (3 oz/90 g) cut-up raw or cooked vegetables 1 medium potato ½ cup (4 fl oz/120 g) vegetable juice
Fruits	4 to 5	1 medium fruit, such as apple or banana 17 grapes ½ cup (3 oz/60 g) fresh, frozen or canned fruit ¼ cup (1½ oz/45 g) dried fruit, such as raisins ¾ cup (6 fl oz/180 mL) 100 percent fruit juice
Fat-free milk and milk products	2 to 3	1 cup (8 fl oz/250 mL) milk or 1 cup or low-fat (8 oz/250 g) yogurt 1½ oz (45 g) cheese 2 cups (16 oz/500 g) low-fat or fat-free cottage cheese

Food group	Daily servings	Serving sizes
Lean meats, poultry and fish	6 or fewer	1 oz (30 g) cooked meats, poultry or fish 1 egg (no more than 4 egg yolks per week)
Nuts, seeds and legumes	4 to 5 a week	⅓ cup (1½ oz/45 g) nuts 2 tablespoons (½ oz/15 g) peanut butter 2 tablespoons (½ oz/15 g) seeds ½ cup (3½ oz/105 g) cooked legumes (dry beans and peas)
Fats and oils	2 to 3	1 teaspoon soft margarine 1 teaspoon vegetable oil 1 tablespoon mayonnaise 2 tablespoons regular salad dressing 4 tablespoons low-fat salad dressing
Sweets and added sugars	5 or fewer a week	1 tablespoon sugar 1 tablespoon jelly or jam ½ cup sorbet or gelatin 1 cup lemonade

These amounts are based on a 2,100-calorie eating plan. Most Americans need between 1,600 and 2,400 calories daily, depending on age, sex and activity level. To lower the number of calories on the DASH diet, see pages 120-121, or talk to a registered dietitian.

The DASH Eating Plan may be found on the National Heart, Lung, and Blood Institute Website at *www.nhlbi.nih.gov.*

The following sections provide more detail on the types of food you may choose when using the DASH diet to help control blood pressure.

Whole grains: 6 to 8 servings. Whole grains include foods such as whole-wheat bread and pasta, oatmeal, brown rice, grits and unsalted popcorn. Whole grains provide more fiber and nutrients than do highly processed or refined grains, such as white rice and white bread. Select plain, whole-grain yeast breads rather than quick breads, sweet rolls or other baked goods that have added fat.

TIP: Breads and pasta are naturally low in fat and calories. To keep a bread slice that way, be cautious about what type of spread you slather on it. Avoid cream and cheese sauces on pasta — opt for vegetable or tomato-based sauces instead.

Vegetables and fruits: 4 to 5 servings each. Eating more vegetables and fruits may be one of the best things you can do to improve your blood pressure and your overall health. In addition to being virtually fat-free and low in calories, vegetables and fruits provide fiber and a variety of wholesome nutrients that help lower blood pressure. Fruits

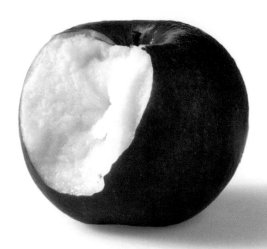

and vegetables also contain phytochemicals, substances that may help reduce your risk of cardiovascular disease and some cancers.

Eating more vegetables and fruits can also help you reduce calories without cutting back on the amount you eat. These foods have a low energy density, meaning there are few calories in a large volume of food — they fill your stomach without adding many pounds. The key is to eat vegetables and fruits plain or with a few herbs and spices and to avoid smothering them with high-fat dips or sauces.

Potatoes, corn and peas make up nearly half the vegetables in the typical American diet. It may be time to think beyond the french fry, and eat more dark green vegetables, such as broccoli, brussels sprouts and spinach. Other nutritious selections include romaine lettuce, tomatoes, bell peppers, onions, carrots and avocados.

Top-rated nutritious fruits include cantaloupe, tangerines, oranges, grapefruit, varieties of berries, apricots, kiwi and watermelon.

TIP: With abundant servings of vegetables, fruits and whole grains, the DASH diet is high in fiber. Increasing your fiber intake can sometimes cause bloating and diarrhea. To avoid these problems, take a gradual approach to increasing your consumption of these foods. You can also try taking Beano, an over-the-counter dietary supplement that helps prevent gas.

Fat-free or low-fat milk and milk products: 2 to 3 servings. Dairy products are sources of the essential mineral calcium as well as vitamin D, which helps your body absorb calcium. Diary products are also valuable sources of protein in your diet.

However, you need to use the low-fat or fat-free varieties of dairy products and avoid whole-fat varieties. At the grocery store, select skim or low-fat (1%) milk and yogurt, and fat-free or

low-fat or reduced-fat cheeses. Look for yogurt and cheese that contains less than 200 mg of sodium per serving.

In recipes, substitute lower fat dairy products, such as skim or low-fat milk, for higher fat items. Note, however, that reduced-fat cream cheese and sour cream are higher in sodium than are their higher fat counterparts, so use them prudently.

TIP: If you're lactose intolerant and have problems digesting dairy products, you may benefit from foods containing the enzyme lactase, which can reduce or prevent the symptoms of lactose intolerance. You can also take lactase tablets before eating the foods.

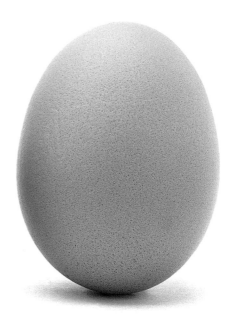

Fish vs. fish oil supplements

Dietitians generally recommend at least two meals of fish every week for possible heart benefits. Some fish — particularly fatty or oily types prevalent in cold water, such as salmon, mackerel, tuna, trout and herring — contain high amounts of omega-3 fatty acids, a type of unsaturated fat. Eating omega-3 fatty acids can reduce your risk of heart disease and help lower blood pressure.

But certain fish contain significant amounts of environmental contaminants, including mercury and polychlorinated biphenyls (PCBs). The amount of toxins depends on the type of fish and where it's caught.

When it comes to a healthy heart, the benefits of eating fish usually outweigh the possible risks of toxic exposure. However, because children and women who are pregnant or considering pregnancy are most susceptible to toxicity in fish, they should limit their consumption.

Some researchers advocate taking fish oil supplements to gain the benefits of omega-3 fatty acids without the risks of toxins. But the American Heart Association recommends fish oil supplements only for people with heart disease or high levels of triglycerides. In high doses, fish oil capsules pose risks, especially if you regularly take aspirin or a blood thinner, such as warfarin (Coumadin). Before you take fish oil capsules, consult your doctor.

To avoid some of the dangers associated with eating fish, follow these guidelines:
- Pay attention to the type of fish you eat and how much you eat. Check with your state or local health department for advisories.
- Eat a variety of fish, including shellfish, canned fish or smaller ocean fish. You can safely eat 12 ounces a week of cooked fish. Avoid large, predatory fish such as shark, swordfish and tilefish.
- Women and children should eat no more than 6 ounces of canned tuna a week and no more than 12 ounces of most other fish.
- Farm-raised salmon has significantly higher levels of PCBs than wild salmon does. But mercury is found equally in farm-raised and wild fish.

Lean meats, poultry and fish: 6 or fewer servings. These foods are rich sources of protein, B vitamins, magnesium, iron and zinc. Choose lean cuts of meat, such as tenderloin, round or sirloin, and trim away the fat. When preparing poultry, remove the skin to reduce fat by about half. Because even lean varieties contain plenty of fat and cholesterol, however, try to limit all animal food sources.

Fish is one of the healthiest animal protein sources. Some fish contain high amounts of omega-3 fatty acids, which can reduce the risk of coronary artery disease and sudden cardiac death and lower blood pressure.

TIP: Choose fresh meat, poultry and fish rather than processed, smoked or cured products. These often contain more than 200 mg of sodium per serving. Broiling, roasting and poaching are the healthiest ways to prepare meat, poultry and fish. You can cook fish in parchment paper or foil to seal in flavor and juices.

Nuts, seeds and legumes: 4 to 5 servings a week. These foods range from almonds, peanuts, walnuts, hazelnuts, peanut butter and sunflower seeds to legumes such as beans, split peas and lentils. They're an excellent source of protein and have no cholesterol. They also provide a variety of nutrients, including magnesium and potassium, plus phytochemicals and fiber. Nuts and seeds contain fat, but most of it is unsaturated, the type that helps protect against coronary artery disease.

TIP: Be careful about salted nuts. Choose products with less than 200 mg of sodium per serving.

Fats and oils: 2 to 3 servings. Many people are surprised to hear that certain fats are essential for good health. Fats provide reserves of stored energy and play vital roles in different body processes. But your consumption of fats should be limited to the monounsaturated varieties. All fats contain approximately 45 calories a serving and are a high-density food. In the DASH studies, 27 percent of calories in the daily diet came from fats, including the fat in or added to food.

Animal products — meat, dairy products and eggs — are the main source of fat in the American diet. Vegetables, fruits and grains are relatively low in fat. Healthy choices of fat include soft margarine and olive, canola, corn and safflower oils.

Choose fats wisely

Not all fats are created equal. Most plans for healthy eating, including the DASH diet, call on you to sharply limit the amount of saturated fat you consume. Foods high in saturated fats include red meat, whole-fat dairy products and tropical oils such as palm and coconut.

Another type of unhealthy fat is trans-fatty acid, which can raise your "bad" LDL cholesterol levels and increase your risk of cardiovascular disease. Trans-fatty acids are found in partially hydrogenated oils, a common ingredient in crackers, cookies and deep-fried foods. Checking food labels can help you steer clear of these bad fats.

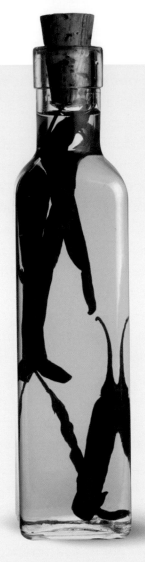

The healthier fats include monounsaturated fats — found in olive oil, canola oil, peanut oil, nuts and avocados — and omega-3 fatty acids. Fatty fish such as salmon, mackerel and herring contain high amounts of omega-3 fatty acids, while smaller amounts are found in green leafy vegetables, soybeans, nuts, flaxseed and canola oil.

Omega-3 fatty acids can benefit your heart by lowering your blood triglyceride level and reducing your risk of blood clots, artery-clogging plaques and sudden death from abnormal heart rhythms. They also lower blood pressure.

TIP: Invest in nonstick pans to cook foods. If you normally add a tablespoon of vegetable oil to a skillet, you can save 120 calories and 14 grams of fat by using a nonstick skillet instead. Vegetable oil cooking spray only adds about 1 gram of fat and few calories.

Sweets: 5 or fewer per week. Sweets are a high source of calories but offer little nutrition. They include candies, cookies, cakes, pies and other desserts. Don't forget the table sugar you add to cereal, fruit and beverages.

You don't have to give up sweets entirely but be smart about what you select and how big of a portion you take. When you do eat sweets, choose low-fat items rather than sugary treats made with oil or butter.

Best choices include fruit-flavored gelatin, fruit punch, angel food cake, jam, honey, maple syrup and sorbet.

TIP: Replace all or part of the sugar in recipes with cinnamon, nutmeg, vanilla and fruit to enhance sweetness.

Chocolate and blood pressure

Research has linked chocolate to lower blood pressure. Cocoa beans contain flavonols, substances thought to enhance the production of nitric oxide in the body, which can improve blood vessel function and blood flow. But you can't eat just any chocolate off the shelf and get the benefits of flavonols. Standard processing techniques have eliminated these natural chemicals from most commercial chocolate products.

Scientists have experimented with ways of processing cocoa beans that don't destroy the flavonols. Still, even the healthiest chocolate adds calories to your diet. People who need to watch their weight might be better off turning to other sources of flavonols, such as apples and tea.

Three important minerals

The DASH diet emphasizes the benefits of three minerals — potassium, calcium and magnesium — that can play a role in managing high blood pressure. Of the three, potassium packs the biggest punch. Studies link a high potassium intake with lower blood pressure, especially in blacks.

The Institute of Medicine recommends that all adult Americans boost their intake of potassium. For most people, the best way to get enough potassium is to eat more potassium-rich foods, such as fruits and vegetables (see page 102.). By eating eight to 10 servings a day of fruits and vegetables, you're more likely to get the recommended potassium intake of 4.7 grams a day. Unfortunately, only about 10 percent of men and less than 1 percent of women consume that amount.

Some people have to be cautious about their potassium intake, however. If you have kidney disease, congestive heart failure or diabetes, talk to your doctor about the levels of potassium and other minerals in your diet.

In addition to the support it provides to your bones and teeth, calcium is also needed for the proper function of your heart, muscles and nerves. And contrary to popular belief, the need for calcium actually increases as you get older. That's because the human body needs a constant replenishment of calcium and, with age, your body will become less efficient at absorbing calcium from the food you eat.

It's recommended that most adults get between 1,000 milligrams (mg) and 1,500 mg of calcium each day (see page 103). Unfortunately, many adults don't consume enough calcium — the typical American diet typically includes only about 600 mg. If you're trying to lose weight, you may need to monitor calcium intake carefully because of your reduced calorie consumption.

Magnesium has many biochemical functions in the body, including helping to maintain a normal heart rhythm. The mineral is found in a wide variety of foods and in drinking water. You can get an adequate amount by regularly eating green leafy vegetables, whole grains, legumes and small amounts of meat, poultry and fish. Nuts and seeds also are good sources of magnesium (see page 103).

What about mineral supplements?

A healthy diet should provide adequate amounts of potassium, calcium and magnesium. Studies indicate that getting these nutrients from foods rather than supplements helps ensure the right mix of the nutrients.

Potassium supplements can have serious side effects. And some blood pressure medications, such as potassium-retaining diuretics, angiotensin-converting enzyme (ACE) inhibitors, angiotensin II receptor blockers and renin inhibitors, can increase potassium levels in your blood. Take potassium supplements only if your doctor recommends them.

If you take a diuretic medication that causes your body to lose potassium, your doctor may recommend a potassium supplement. Calcium and magnesium supplements generally aren't required to control high blood pressure.

The shakedown on salt

Of all the issues related to high blood pressure, none has been more heavily debated than salt — specifically, the sodium in salt. The research on sodium reveals a complicated picture. And in the real world, just saying no to salt is not so easy or straightforward.

Despite the controversy, study results continue to support limiting sodium as a means to lower blood pressure. The effects of a lower sodium intake are greater for people with high blood pressure, older adults, African-Americans and people with diabetes or long-term kidney disease. But moderating salt consumption can benefit anyone, regardless of age, race, sex or health status.

Sources of potassium, calcium and magnesium

Mineral	How it works	Where it's found
Potassium	Balances the amount of sodium in your cells; high intake reduces blood pressure	Many fruits and vegetables, whole grains, legumes, dairy products, potatoes

Good sources of potassium include:

Apricots, bananas, cantaloupe, cherries, dates, figs, honeydew, kiwi, mango, nectarine, orange, papaya, prunes and tangerines, apple juice, grapefruit juice, grape juice, orange juice, pineapple juice, artichokes, beans (dried), beets, broccoli, brussels sprouts, collard greens or kohlrabi (cooked), mushrooms, parsley, potatoes, pumpkin, spinach, squash, zucchini, cocoa mix (powder), milk (fat-free or low-fat), peanut butter, tofu, yogurt (fat-free or low-fat)

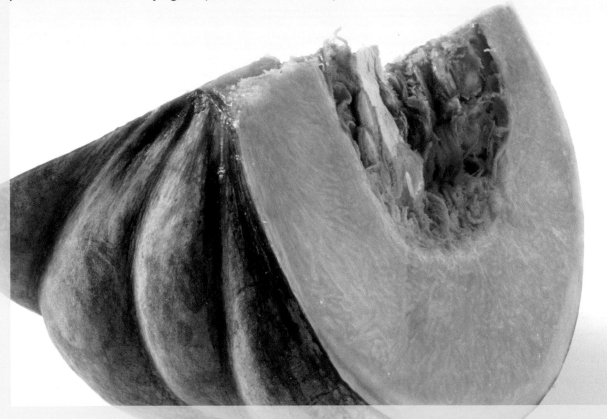

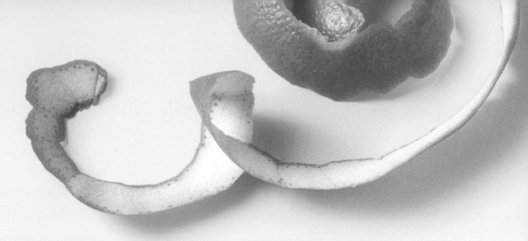

Mineral	How it works	Where it's found
Calcium	Not proved to prevent high blood pressure, but eating too little is linked with high blood pressure	Dairy products, green leafy vegetables, fish with edible bones, calcium-fortified foods

Good sources of calcium include:

Milk (fat-free or low-fat), tofu set with calcium, yogurt (fat-free or low-fat), orange juice (calcium-fortified), cereal (calcium-fortified), canned salmon with bones, mozzarella cheese (part-skim), collard greens (cooked), bread (calcium-fortified), cottage cheese (low-fat), navy beans (cooked), broccoli (cooked)

Mineral	How it works	Where it's found
Magnesium	Deficient levels are linked with higher blood pressure	Legumes, green leafy vegetables, nuts and seeds, whole grains, lean meats

Good sources of magnesium include:

Good sources of magnesium include a wide variety of foods as well as drinking water. Foods include green leafy vegetables, whole grains, legumes, nuts and seeds, and even small amounts of meat, poultry and fish.

Sodium's role

An essential mineral, sodium helps maintain the right balance of fluids in your body. It also helps transmit nerve impulses and influences the contraction and relaxation of muscles.

You get sodium from the foods you eat. Many foods naturally contain sodium, but about 77 percent of your intake comes from compounds added to food during commercial processing and about 11 percent from meal preparation at home — added during cooking or while eating. What's known as table salt, which is a compound of sodium and chloride, is the most common source of sodium.

Recommended sodium intake is 1,500 mg a day, with an upper limit of 2,400 mg for most healthy adults. Most Americans consume much more than that — the estimated average daily sodium intake for Americans ranges from 3,100 to 4,700 mg.

Your kidneys regulate the amount of sodium in your body. When sodium levels fall, your kidneys conserve sodium. When levels are high, the kidneys flush out the excess amount of sodium through your urine. Genetic factors as well as heart, kidney, liver and lung diseases all can interfere with your ability to regulate sodium.

When your kidneys can't eliminate enough sodium, the mineral starts to accumulate in your blood. Because sodium attracts and holds water, your blood volume increases. Your heart has to work harder to move the increased volume of blood, increasing the pressure on your arteries. Chemicals in your body that influence the sodium balance are also affected.

Sodium sensitivity

How people's bodies react to sodium varies. Some healthy adults — including some with high blood pressure — can consume as much sodium as they like with little or no effect on their blood pressure.

For others, too much sodium quickly leads to higher blood pressure, often triggering chronic high blood pressure. This response is referred to as sodium sensitivity or salt sensitivity.

Approximately 60 percent of Americans with high blood pressure and 25 percent of Americans with normal blood pressure are sodium sensitive. The condition is more common in blacks and older adults. In addition, people with diabetes or long-term kidney disease tend to be more sensitive to high levels of sodium.

Exactly what causes sodium sensitivity isn't known, but genetic factors likely affect the way your body handles salt. The sensitivity can be passed down through families, and researchers have identified several genes associated with higher blood pressure (as well as lower blood pressure).

There's no easy way to tell if you're sodium sensitive. Some researchers have developed blood tests that can detect salt sensitivity, but more studies are needed to confirm their reliability. If it's determined that you have a sensitivity to salt, following a low-sodium diet should produce a noticeable reduction in blood pressure.

Reducing sodium is important for another reason. At least one study found that sodium sensitivity increases your risk of death due to heart disease and other health-related causes,

whether or not you have high blood pressure. In addition to increasing your blood pressure, sodium sensitivity can increase your risk of kidney problems and cardiovascular disease.

The controversy

Ever since the recommendation 30 years ago that all Americans — not just those with hypertension — limit sodium to control blood pressure, the issue has sparked controversy. While this action helps some individuals, it's also true that when others cut back on sodium, their blood pressure decreases very little, if at all.

Critics point out that studies linking a low-sodium diet to lower blood pressure don't show improvements in actual outcomes — in other words, the studies don't prove that a low-sodium diet results in fewer deaths from conditions associated with high blood pressure such as heart disease and stroke. These researchers also raise concerns that a low-sodium diet may actually increase the risk of higher blood fats and increased insulin resistance.

Many large studies, however, indicate that when people consume less sodium, their blood pressure will fall and, furthermore, fewer deaths occur from heart attack and stroke. This suggests that, while limiting sodium may benefit some individuals minimally, it has a major impact on the general population in preventing high blood pressure and reducing death and disability.

Even a small reduction in average blood pressure across a large population — perhaps just 2 mm Hg in pressure — can lead to significant positive outcomes for the overall health and well being of that population.

The American Heart Association, the American Medical Association and various U.S. government agencies continue to monitor scientific information about sodium and blood pressure. Their positions support limiting sodium as a reasonable and safe expedient to good health.

One thing that the DASH studies and other research makes clear is that limiting sodium works best in the context of an overall healthy diet. Various aspects of your diet can affect blood pressure. For example, losing weight and eating a healthy diet — combined with low sodium intake — are more effective in managing high blood pressure than limiting sodium alone.

Current recommendations

The National High Blood Pressure Education Program, sponsored by the National Institutes of Health, recommends that all Americans, including children and teens, limit sodium to less than 2,400 mg a day. That's equivalent to what's contained in about a teaspoon of salt.

If you have high blood pressure, your doctor may advise eating even less sodium. Making sure you get enough potassium will help further to control your sodium levels.

Many health professionals and organizations, including Mayo Clinic, support a lower sodium diet. Here's why:
- If you have high blood pressure, reducing sodium can lower your blood pressure. Limiting sodium in combination with other lifestyle changes may be enough to keep you from having to take medication to control your blood pressure.
- If you're taking blood pressure medication, limiting sodium can help increase the effectiveness of the drug. Even if you're taking a diuretic, it's still important to reduce sodium in your diet.

Sodium-based food additives

These compounds that contain sodium are commonly added to food during processing and cooking.

- **Baking powder.** A mixture of baking soda, starch and an acid used to leaven quick breads and cakes.
- **Baking soda (sodium bicarbonate).** Sometimes used to leaven breads and cakes; sometimes added to vegetables in cooking; used as an alkalizer for indigestion.
- **Disodium phosphate.** Present in some quick-cooking cereals and processed cheeses.
- **Monosodium glutamate (MSG).** Flavor enhancer used in home and restaurant cooking and in many packaged, canned and frozen foods.
- **Salt (sodium chloride).** Used in cooking or at the table; used in canning and preserving.
- **Sodium alginate.** Used in many chocolate milks and ice creams to make a smooth mixture.
- **Sodium benzoate.** Used as a preservative in many condiments, such as relishes, sauces and salad dressings.
- **Sodium hydroxide.** Used in food processing to soften and loosen skins of ripe olives and certain fruits and vegetables.
- **Sodium nitrate.** Used in cured meats and sausages.
- **Sodium propionate.** Used in pasteurized cheese and in some breads and cakes to inhibit growth of molds.
- **Sodium sulfite.** Used to bleach certain fruits, such as maraschino cherries and glazed or crystallized fruits that are to be artificially colored; used as a preservative in some dried fruits, such as prunes.

Source: American Heart Association, Sodium and Blood Pressure, © 1996.
Reprinted with permission.

- If you're at risk of high blood pressure, limiting sodium and making other lifestyle changes may prevent its development.
- If you don't have high blood pressure, limiting sodium is still a safe and reasonable action. In addition, it may lower your risk of high blood pressure as you get older. Many doctors say that curbing salt intake should begin in childhood, to help prevent blood pressure related problems that may begin as early as the teen years.

The challenge of eating less salt

If your doctor or registered dietitian has suggested that you cut back on sodium to lower your blood pressure, it's advice that you should follow. Even if you haven't been told to reduce sodium, try to moderate the amount you eat each day.

Of course, that's easier said than done. Research shows that reducing salt in your diet is notoriously difficult. Salt makes food taste good and it acts as a preservative.

Many doctors believe that the real problem isn't overuse of the saltshaker but rather the hidden salt added to processed foods. More than three-fourths of the salt people consume comes from processed foods rather than salt added at the table.

Many commercially prepared foods, snack foods, fast foods and restaurant foods contain far more sodium than you need. For example, a serving of canned chicken soup may have about 1,100 mg of sodium, while a cheese Danish may have 750 mg. As consumers increasingly rely on convenience and ready-to-eat foods, responsibility for sodium intake falls more and more on the food industry.

For this reason, some doctors are emphasizing a public health approach to lowering sodium intake, in addition to advocating changes in individual behavior.

The American Medical Association (AMA) and the American Public Health Association have called on food companies and restaurants to voluntarily limit sodium levels in foods by 50 percent by 2016. The AMA wants the Food and Drug Administration to require food labels to carry warnings on any foods that contains more than 480 mg of sodium per serving.

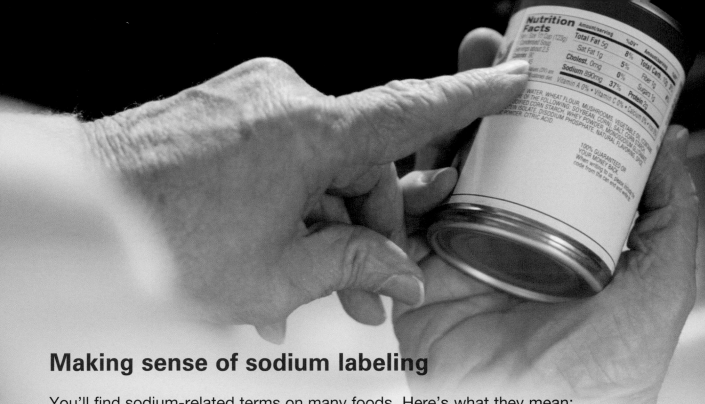

Making sense of sodium labeling

You'll find sodium-related terms on many foods. Here's what they mean:

- **Sodium-free or salt-free.** Each serving in this product contains less than 5 mg of sodium.
- **Very low sodium.** Each serving contains 35 mg of sodium or less.
- **Low sodium.** Each serving contains 140 mg of sodium or less.
- **Reduced or less sodium.** The product contains at least 25 percent less sodium than the regular version.
- **Lite or light in sodium.** The sodium content has been reduced by at least 50 percent from the regular version.
- **Unsalted or no salt added**. No salt is added during processing of a food that normally contains salt. However, some foods with these labels may still be high in sodium.

Don't be fooled — foods labeled "reduced sodium" or "light in sodium" may still contain a lot of salt. If the regular product starts out high in sodium, reducing it by 25 percent or 50 percent may make little difference. For example, regular canned chicken noodle soup contains about 1,100 mg of sodium per cup, while the reduced-sodium version may still have 820 mg per cup. The bottom line? Read the labels carefully.

Spice it up

It's easy to make food taste good without using salt. Try these suggestions for herbs, spices and flavorings to enhance the taste of various foods. Here's an extra tip: Place dried herbs in a little liquid a few minutes before adding them to a recipe to help release flavors.

Meat, poultry, fish

Beef
: Bay leaf, dry mustard, horseradish, marjoram, nutmeg, onion, pepper, sage, thyme

Chicken
: Basil and tomatoes, dill, ginger, oregano, paprika, parsley, rosemary, sage, tarragon, thyme

Fish
: Bay leaf, curry powder, dill, dry mustard, lemon juice, paprika

Lamb
: Cranberry, curry powder, garlic, rosemary

Pork
: Cranberry, garlic, onion, oregano, pepper, sage

Veal
: Bay leaf, curry powder, ginger, oregano

Vegetables

Broccoli
: Lemon juice, oregano

Carrots
: Cinnamon, honey, nutmeg, orange juice, rosemary, sage

Cauliflower
: Nutmeg, tarragon

Corn
: Chives, cumin, fresh tomatoes, green pepper, paprika, parsley

Green beans
: Dill, lemon juice, nutmeg, tarragon, unsalted French dressing

Peas
: Mint, onion, parsley

Potatoes
: Dill, garlic, green pepper, onion, parsley, sage

Tomatoes
: Basil, dill, onion, oregano, parsley, sage

Low-sodium soups

Creamed
: Bay leaf, dill, paprika, peppercorns, tarragon

Vegetable
: Basil, bay leaf, curry, dill, garlic, onion, oregano

Other

Popcorn
: Curry, garlic powder, onion powder

Rice
: Basil, cumin, curry, green pepper, oregano

Salads
: Basil, dill, lemon juice, parsley, vinegar

? How long will it take to get over my cravings for salt?

It will take your taste buds several weeks to several months to fully adjust to the taste of food prepared with less salt. But if you persevere, highly salted food will soon begin to taste unpleasant. Salt substitutes may help you taper down but use them with care (see page 113).

Here's another dietary example: To reduce fat intake, many people have switched from whole milk to skim milk. When they first made the switch, skim milk probably seemed tasteless and watered down. But as they adjusted to skim, they found that whole milk products began to taste too thick and rich.

Public health officials suggest that by slowly reducing the salt in processed foods, people will adjust to the lower salt taste. This practice is already under way in countries such as England.

Limiting sodium intake is challenging — but small changes can bring positive results. As you decrease your salt use gradually, your taste buds will have time to adjust and your preference for sodium will lessen, allowing you to enjoy the taste of the food itself. Most people find that a few weeks after reducing salt, they no longer miss it.

The following steps can help you reduce the amount of salt and sodium in your diet:

Eat more fresh foods. Fresh produce such as vegetables and fruits naturally contain less sodium than do processed foods. The canned vegetables and vegetable juices that you bring home from the store usually have added salt.

Fresh meat is lower in sodium than smoked or cured meats, such as luncheon meat, bacon, hot dogs, sausage and ham. These foods have sodium added for flavor and to help preserve them. Some fresh meats also have salt injected into them and may be labeled "Flavor enhanced with saline solution." Check the Nutrition Facts label and avoid meats with more than 200 mg of sodium per serving.

Soups, frozen dinners, sauces, mixes and other instant products typically have added salt. Snacks such as potato chips, corn chips, pretzels, popcorn, crackers and nuts often contain a large amount of added salt. It's best to eat them sparingly. Choose fresh fruits and raw vegetables for snacking, and buy unsalted nuts and seeds.

Choose lower sodium products. Some processed foods that are high in sodium are also prepared in lower sodium versions, often labeled as "low salt" or "low sodium." These include soups, broths, canned vegetables, processed lean meats, ketchup and soy sauce. Just because a food is low in fat or calories doesn't mean it's low in sodium. Sometimes extra sodium is added to low-fat products to enhance flavor.

Read labels. The Nutrition Facts label tells you how much sodium is in each serving. Choose foods with under 200 mg of sodium per serving. Generally,

any product with 5 percent of the Daily Value for sodium per serving is low and 20 percent is high.

Some over-the-counter drugs contain large amounts of sodium. They include some antacids, alkalizers, laxatives and cough medicines. If you use such a product often, check the label or ask a pharmacist about its sodium content.

Don't add salt when cooking. Cook rice, pasta and hot cereals without adding salt. Remove salt from recipes whenever possible — a dash of salt contains ⅛ teaspoon (300 mg) of sodium. You can combine a no-salt product with a regular product in some recipes. For instance, if your recipe calls for 16 ounces of tomato sauce, use 8 ounces of no-salt-added sauce and 8 ounces regular sauce.

Don't add salt at the table. Don't salt food before you've tasted it. If you think your food needs more flavor, try another seasoning, such as lemon, pepper or a sodium-free herb blend. If you have a favorite seasoning blend that contains salt, look at the ingredients to see what's flavoring it besides salt and try to find an alternative. For example, use garlic or onion powder rather than garlic or onion salt.

Rinse canned foods. Rinsing canned vegetables and meats helps remove some of the sodium, but don't consider this to be a great way to reduce sodium in your diet. In fact, it only removes about one-third of the sodium. It's best to use fresh or frozen vegetables.

Limit your use of condiments. Salad dressings, sauces, dips, ketchup, mustard and relish all contain a high amount of sodium, as do pickles and olives. Make your meals more flavorful with herbs, spices, garlic powder, onion powder and pepper, unsalted ketchup, mustard and barbecue sauce, lemon juice, flavoring extracts and vinegar, prepared horseradish and table wine (not cooking wine).

About salt substitutes. Before you try a salt substitute, check with your doctor. Some contain a mixture of sodium chloride (salt) and other compounds. To achieve that familiar salty taste, you may end up using more of the salt substitute than you would regular salt.

In addition, potassium chloride is a common ingredient in salt substitutes and some "low sodium" products such as broth or bouillon. Too much potassium can be harmful if you have kidney problems or you're taking certain med-

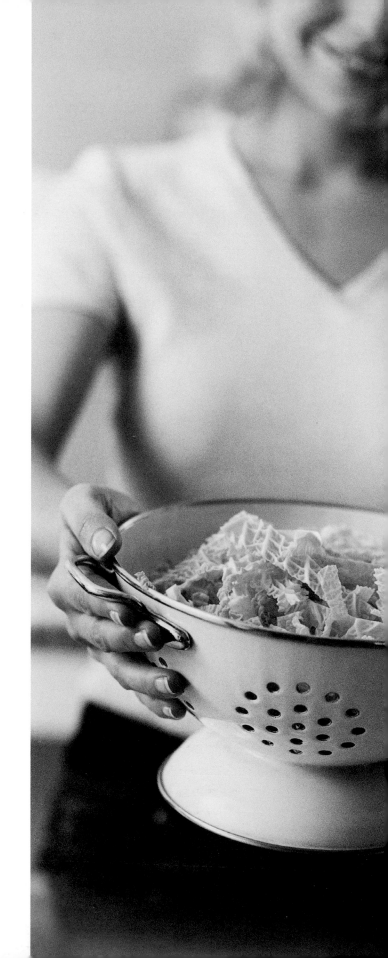

ications, such as a potassium-sparing diuretic, to treat high blood pressure or heart failure.

Remove salt from kosher meats. To kosher meat without using salt, broil the meat on a flat pan that allows the juices to run off. To remove salt in kosher meats, place the raw meat in a large pot filled with cold water and bring the pot to a boil. Then remove the pot from the heat and drain the water. Most of the salt will drain away.

Your sodium guide

The following guide is meant to complement the DASH diet. It lists foods that are low in sodium and can be eaten frequently.

Whole grains and starches
- Whole-grain bread, rolls and cereals with less than 200 mg of sodium in a serving
- Quick breads such as pancakes or biscuits made from home recipes that use no buttermilk and little or no salt
- Potatoes, rice and pasta
- Unsalted popcorn, pretzels, chips and crackers
- Low-sodium canned soups, bouillon and broth

Vegetables
- Fresh, unsalted frozen or low-sodium canned vegetables
- No-salt-added or low-sodium tomato juice and vegetable juice
- No-salt-added canned tomato products

Fruits
- Fresh and frozen fruit and canned fruit in juice or water

Dairy products
- Fat-free or low-fat milk, cottage cheese and yogurt
- Reduced-fat cheeses with less than 200 mg of sodium per ounce

Limit (2-3 times a week):
- Regular cottage cheese and aged natural cheese such as brick cheese, Monterey Jack and mild cheddar

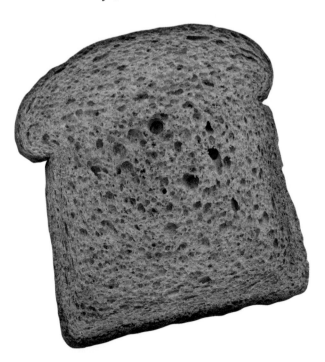

Beverages
- Bottled water and beverages with less than 70 mg of sodium in a serving
- Tap water (Sodium content varies with the local water supply.)

Limit (1-2 servings a day):
- Alcoholic beverages
- Coffee and tea
- Cocoa (made with cocoa powder)

Lean meats, poultry, & fish
- Fresh or frozen meat and poultry without added salt or saline
- Fresh or frozen fish and shellfish (unbreaded and not packed in brine or with added sodium)
- Water-packed canned tuna or other seafood; canned salmon with no added salt
- Egg whites

Limit (2-3 times a week):
- Canned tuna and other canned seafood packed with 50 percent to 60 percent less salt than usual
- Reduced-sodium processed meats and cheeses
- Lobster and crab

Main dish items
- Homemade dishes and soups without added salt or canned vegetables as ingredients
- Frozen and microwave dinners that have less than 600 mg of sodium in a dinner

Nuts, seeds, and legumes
- Low-sodium or no-salt-added peanut butter
- Unsalted nuts and seeds
- Dried peas, beans and lentils

Fats and oils (*use sparingly*)
- Oil, margarine or butter
- Salad dressings with less than 200 mg of sodium in a serving
- Mayonnaise and unsalted gravy
- Cream cheese and sour cream

Desserts and sweets (*use sparingly*)
- Homemade desserts, cooked pudding and box mixes with less than 200 mg sodium in a serving
- Fresh fruit, gelatin, fruit ice, sherbet, plain cake, meringue, ice cream and frozen yogurt
- Jams, jellies, honey, hard candy and jelly beans

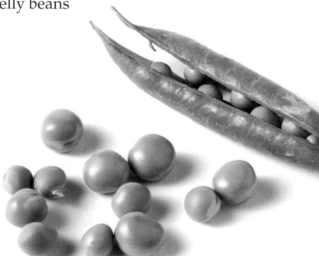

Fresh approach to shopping

Success with the DASH diet starts with the foods you buy. When you're shopping, think fresh and unprocessed. Try to spend most of your time in the produce section, where you can stock up on fruits and vegetables. Here are other tips for healthier shopping with the DASH diet in mind:

Plan. Decide on the meals you're going to make during the coming week and write the ingredients you need on a grocery list. Don't forget about what you'll need for breakfast and snacks. Include plenty of fruits, vegetables, whole-grain breads and cereals on your list. Consider legumes such as lentil or kidney beans as your source of protein.

Buy fresh. Fresh foods are usually better than ready-to-eat foods because you can control what ingredients go into your meals. Fresh foods generally have more flavor, color and health-promoting vitamins, minerals and fiber than do their packaged counterparts. Note that the freshest and healthiest foods tend to be located around the perimeter of a grocery store.

How do I plan a weekly menu?

Set aside time each week to plan menus for the next seven days. That way, you'll have all the ingredients on hand before you start preparing meals. If you know how many calories you should eat each day, the serving recommendations for each food group will guide your decisions.

- Keep menus practical and simple. But at the same time, don't exclude good flavor and fun. Remember that you need to enjoy your meals along with eating healthier. It's OK to include favorite foods, but you may need to adapt the recipes to make them healthier.
- Aim for balance. Try to include at least one serving from most food groups in most meals.
- Don't make meat the focus. Build the main part of your meal around vegetables and fruits, in addition to rice, noodles and other grains.
- Be flexible. Don't get hung up on exact daily serving totals. If on one day you don't reach your target for fruit servings, you can add an extra serving on the next day.

Don't shop on an empty stomach. It's hard to resist the bright packaging and enticing smells of many snack items. To reduce the temptation, go shopping after you've eaten a good meal. If you find yourself shopping when you're hungry, buy a piece of fresh fruit to munch on while you're in the store.

Read the labels. Take time to read food labels on products before purchasing them. The labels inform you about which foods are healthy, and warn you about those that aren't so healthy. They also can help you compare the ingredients of similar foods and select items that are the most nutritious.

Nutrition Facts

Serving Size 1 cup (53g)
Servings Per Container About 8

Amount Per Serving

Calories 190   Calories from Fat 25

	% Daily Value*
Total Fat 3g	5%
Saturated Fat 0g	0%
Trans Fat 0g	
Cholesterol 0mg	0%
Sodium 95mg	4%
Potassium 300mg	9%
Total Carbohydrate 36g	12%
Dietary Fiber 8g	32%
Sugars 13g	
Protein 9g	18%
Vitamin A	0%
Vitamin C	0%
Calcium	4%
Iron	10%

* Percent Daily Values are based on a 2,000 calorie diet. Your Daily Values may be higher or lower depending on your calorie needs.

	Calories:	2,000	2,500
Total Fat	Less than	65g	80g
Sat Fat	Less than	20g	25g
Cholesterol	Less than	300mg	300mg
Sodium	Less than	2,400mg	2,400mg
Total Carbohydrate		300g	375g
Dietary Fiber		25g	30g

Food label example

This example provides a breakdown of calories, fat, carbohydrates, protein, vitamins and minerals in a single serving.

How to read food labels

For more than a decade, packaged goods sold in the United States have carried the Nutrition Facts label. The labels provide valuable information that helps you fit different kinds of food into your eating plan. These labels may seem confusing at first, but once you learn how to interpret them, they make it easier to plan your meals and to comparison shop.

Each Nutrition Facts label contains information based on a single serving of the contents. This information includes:

Serving size. The label indicates the quantity that's considered a single serving and how many servings are in the container. If you eat more or less than the indicated serving, you would need to adjust the calorie and nutrient information accordingly.

Calories from fat. This information allows you to add up the amount of fat you eat and to compare the fat content of different products. Try to limit fat to about 65 grams a day. This amount keeps fat at the recommended level — less than 30 percent of your daily calories, based on a 2,000-calorie diet.

Percent Daily Value. These percentages indicate how much of the recommended daily amounts are in one serving of food, based on a 2,000-calorie diet. In the food label example, one serving provides 300 mg of potassium, or 9 percent of the Daily Value.

For fat, saturated fat and cholesterol, choose foods with a low Percent Daily Value. For total carbohydrate, dietary fiber, vitamins and minerals, try to reach a higher Percent Daily Value.

Sodium. Most sodium that Americans consume comes from processed foods, so it's important to choose foods with less than 200 mg of sodium in a serving, or under 8 percent of the Daily Value. This food label is a good example, but it's not always easy to find products with low sodium content.

Eating smart for weight control

If you're overweight, losing even a few pounds can improve your blood pressure. Losing weight brings other health benefits as well, such as a reduced risk of diabetes and heart disease.

The most successful method for losing weight is to change your eating and activity habits and to slim down gradually. You can accomplish this with the DASH eating plan and regular exercise program. You can modify the plan to lower your calorie levels.

Just because the task may seem daunting doesn't mean that you shouldn't try it — and keep trying to control your weight. Many people have successfully changed their eating and activity habits to maintain weight loss.

Your efforts can pay off for a lifetime. Not only does losing weight lower your blood pressure but studies also show that the effect can last for many years as you keep the weight off.

A little can mean a lot

What is a healthy weight? It's not essential that you become thin. But you can aim for achieving or maintaining a weight that improves your blood pressure and also lessens your risks of other health problems.

Losing as little as 10 pounds may reduce your blood pressure to a healthier level. If you're overweight, reducing your weight by 5 percent to 10 percent may be a good goal. Once you've achieved that goal, you can try for another 5 percent to 10 percent if you need to lose more weight. Over time, these losses can add up to a significant improvement in your health.

The DASH diet and weight loss

If you're planning to lose weight, you'll probably need to consume fewer calories than you consume now (and burn more calories through exercise).

To lower the standard DASH eating plan from a calorie level of 2,100 to 1,600 per day, use these serving guidelines:

Food groups	Daily servings
Whole grains	6
Vegetables	3 to 4
Fruits	4
Fat-free or low-fat milk and milk products	2 to 3
Lean meats, poultry, fish	3 to 6
Nuts, seeds, legumes	3 a week
Fats and oils	2
Sweets and added sugars	0

Source: National Heart, Lung, and Blood Institute, DASH Eating Plan, 2006

To trim calories from the DASH diet, start by replacing higher calorie foods with more fruits and vegetables. This also helps your blood pressure control. Here are other ways to cut calories from your eating plan.

- Pay attention to energy density. Some foods pack a lot of calories into a small portion — they're energy dense. Other foods, such as fruits and vegetables, have fewer calories in a greater volume. When you choose foods that have a low energy density, you can eat more while consuming fewer calories.
- Prepare stews, casseroles and stir-fries with half the meat the recipe calls for, adding extra vegetables or tofu instead. For example, instead of 5 ounces of chicken, prepare a stir-fry with 2 ounces of chicken and 1½ cups of vegetables. Use a small amount of vegetable oil.
- Use fat-free or low-fat condiments.
- Limit foods with added sugar, such as candy bars, pie, flavored yogurts, regular soft drinks and ice cream.
- Don't forget about the calories in beverages, including juice, alcohol and coffee with milk, sugar, cocoa or whipping cream.
- Sauté onions, mushrooms or other vegetables in a small amount of water instead of butter or oil.
- Grill, broil, poach, roast or stir-fry foods instead of frying them.

Calculating calories

Here's an easy way to figure out how many calories you can eat in a day and still lose an average of 1 pound (0.5 kilogram) a week:

_____ x 10 = _____
(current weight in pounds)   (daily calories)

or

_____ x 22 = _____
(current weight in kilograms)   (daily calories)

Use this calorie level as your daily target.

Eating well when eating out

A trip to the restaurant can be a mine-field of temptations. The sights and smells of food tantalize your senses. Your best intentions crumble before the menu items that beckon to you.

In fact, you *can* eat nutritiously away from home. You need to be more menu savvy to healthy choices. And be mind-ful of two common eating-out challenges: the urge to order more food than you need and the impulse to eat every bit of food on your plate, even when the portion sizes are too large.

When an entree is larger than you want — which is more often than not — ask if you can have the lunch portion, even if you're eating dinner. You can also request a take-home bag when the meal is served. Or you might choose an appetizer for an entree or split a meal with a companion.

Hidden calories refer to the extra calories added to many dishes that come from ingredients you may not be aware of. That's why they're such a problem when you're trying to lose weight.

Ingredients are often added to enhance the flavor, color or texture of food — for example, seasonings, sauces or dressings. And sometimes they're part of the preparation process — for example, oil or butter used in cooking. These calories add up in subtle ways.

What to order

When reviewing a restaurant menu, use these guidelines to help you keep your eating plan on target:

Appetizer. Choose appetizers with fresh vegetables, fruit or fish. Avoid fried or breaded appetizers.

Soup. You're often better off avoiding soup and choosing fruit or a salad. Broth- or tomato-based soups are often high in sodium. Creamed soups, chowders, puréed soups and some fruit soups contain heavy cream and egg yolks and may also be high in sodium.

Salad. Order a lettuce or spinach salad with the dressing on the side, and limit yourself to one soupspoon of dressing. Try olive oil with vinegar for a salad topping. Caesar salads and chef salads are high in fat, cholesterol and sodium. Taco salads aren't good choices because they contain high-fat, high-sodium items such as cheese, guacamole, ground beef and a fried shell.

Bread. If you're offered a bread basket, choose whole-grain bread, rolls, breadsticks or bagels. Eat them plain or with a little honey, jam or jelly. These fat-free toppings contribute few calories when used sparingly. Muffins, garlic toast and croissants have more fat. Crackers can be high in sodium and fat.

Entree. Look for entrees with descriptions that indicate low-fat content, such as London broil, grilled chicken breast, baked or poached fish or broiled beef or chicken kebobs.

Avoid items with descriptions indicating higher fat content, such as prime rib of beef, veal parmigiana, stuffed shrimp, fried chicken, filet mignon with bearnaise sauce, creamed vegetables and cream sauces.

If you're not sure how much fat is in a sauce, ask for it on the side so that you can control how much you add.

Side dish. Choose a baked potato, boiled new potatoes, steamed vegetables, rice or fresh fruit instead of french fries, hash browns, twice-baked potatoes, potato chips, onion rings or mayonnaise-based salads, such as potato salad. Ask that no butter, margarine or salt be used to prepare the dish.

Condiments. Choose items such as fresh tomato, cucumber and lettuce for your sandwiches. Avoid olives, pickles and sauerkraut, and use ketchup, mustard and mayonnaise sparingly.

Dessert. Choose fresh fruit, poached spiced fruit, plain cake with fruit purée, or sorbet or sherbet.

Alcohol. Alcohol is high in calories. Excessive alcohol consumption can also raise your blood pressure. If you choose to drink alcohol, limit the amount to one drink a day if you're a woman and one or two drinks if you're a man. Alcohol's relationship to high blood pressure is discussed in greater detail in Step 3 of this book.

Eating out isn't a time to forget all you know about choosing healthy foods. In fact, dining out can be a great time to try different cuisines. But the same eating principles apply to your decisions.

Many restaurants provide healthy choices. Some restaurants even reserve a special section of their menu for healthier fare. Many restaurants will honor special requests to prepare an item with less fat and sodium.

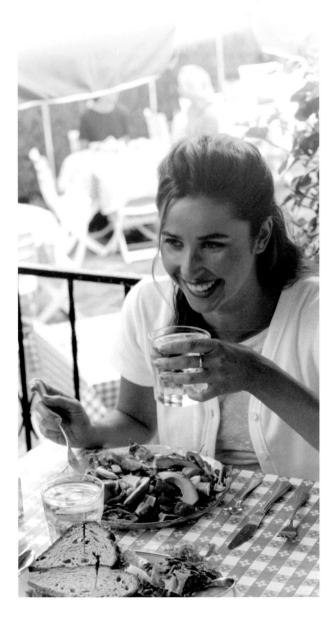

Putting it in perspective

If the myriad of suggestions in this chapter seems overwhelming, remember that eating well isn't an all-or-nothing proposition. Each food you eat doesn't have to be perfect. Perfection isn't the goal — being persistent in your pursuit of healthy eating is what's most important.

Over time, this approach to eating well will become a habit that will help you manage your high blood pressure, improve your health, control your weight and feel better about yourself, as well.

Wrap-up

Key points to remember:
- A healthy diet can reduce your blood pressure as much as some medications.
- The DASH diet can help lower your blood pressure by promoting vegetables, fruits and whole grain products. The diet is low in sodium and fat and high in minerals such as potassium, calcium and magnesium.
- Sodium can significantly increase blood pressure if you have sodium sensitivity.
- Whether you have high blood pressure or not, limiting sodium to less than 2,400 mg daily is reasonable and safe.
- Blood pressure generally increases with weight gain and decreases with weight loss. Losing as few as 10 pounds can help lower your pressure.
- The best approach to slow, steady weight loss is based on eating nutritious foods and getting regular physical activity.

Step 2

Get regular exercise

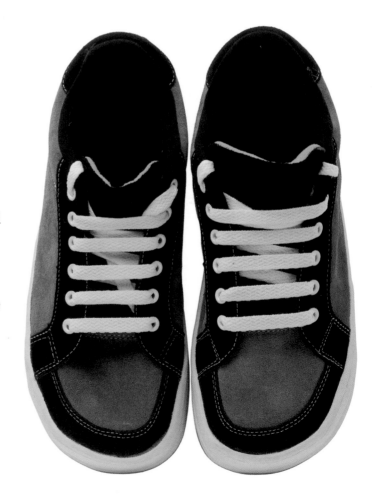

Being physically active, in combination with healthy eating, is vital for reducing and controlling your blood pressure. Regular activity can lower your blood pressure by about the same amount as many blood pressure medications can.

Conversely, one reason why high blood pressure is so common may be that people aren't active enough. Modern conveniences and a shortage of free time have caused Americans to become increasingly sedentary.

According to data from the National Health Interview Survey (2005), only 24 percent of Americans age 18 and older participated in three or more periods (10 minutes or more) of vigorous leisure-time activity a week. And 62 percent of Americans got no regular leisure-time physical activity at all.

Using physical activity to help lower your blood pressure doesn't mean spending long hours at the gym. It's not necessary to live by the motto of "No pain, no gain," pushing yourself to your limits of endurance. It's enough that you remain committed and make every effort to include physical activity in your daily routine.

Moderate activity can be very beneficial to your cardiovascular health and to your overall health. A key element to receiving these benefits, however, is that you exercise with regularity. A way to do that is finding activities that are interesting and enjoyable.

Benefits of regular activity

Physical activity is important for controlling blood pressure because it makes your heart stronger. With greater strength, your heart is able to pump more blood with less effort. And the more efficient your heart is at pumping blood, the less force will need to be exerted on your arteries.

Regular physical activity can lower your blood pressure by 5 to 10 millimeters of mercury (mm Hg). If you're at risk of high blood pressure, that's low enough to keep the condition from ever developing. If you have high blood pressure, a slight reduction may be enough to prevent you from having to take medication. If you're taking medication, it's enough to make your medication work more effectively.

Being physically active can improve your health in a variety of ways. In addition to helping control blood pressure, regular activity also reduces your risk of heart attack, high cholesterol, diabetes, osteoporosis and some cancers. It gives you more energy, improves your mood, and helps you to sleep better and to manage stress.

In addition, regular activity helps promote weight loss. When you gain weight, your blood pressure often increases. And when you lose weight, your blood pressure often goes down. The most successful method of losing weight includes doing regular activity of moderate intensity on most days of the week.

Physical activity vs. exercise

The terms *physical activity* and *exercise* are closely related — and often overlap — but there's a difference. Physical activity refers to any body movement that burns calories, such as raking leaves or taking the dog for a walk. Exercise is a more structured form of physical activity. It generally involves repetitive movements that strengthen or develop a part of your body and improve your cardio-vascular fitness. Exercise includes walking, swimming and biking.

Therefore, exercise is a form of physical activity, but not all physical activity fits the definition of exercise. Either way, the good news is that many health benefits may be gained through regular physical activity, even if it's not in a structured, repetitive form.

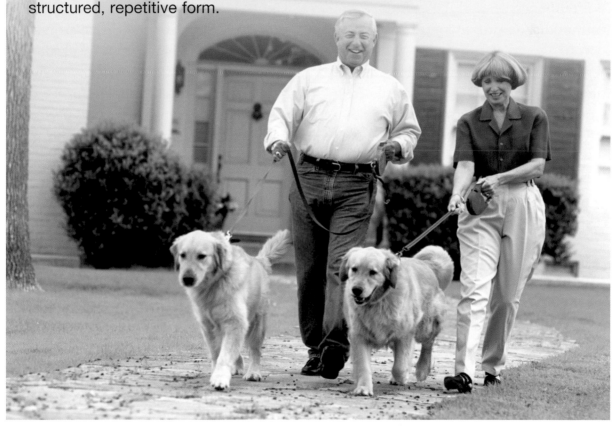

Activity vs. intensity

For many years, the belief was that you had to exercise vigorously to be physically fit and to improve your health. As a result, people developed an all-or-nothing attitude toward exercise. And this led to a high dropout rate.

But studies show that light activity is also good for your blood pressure and overall health — and it's definitely better than doing nothing at all.

In 2002, the Department of Health and Human Services issued guidelines urging Americans to take part in regular physical activity. These guidelines recommend a minimum of one of the following options:

- 30 to 60 minutes of moderate activity on at least five days a week
- 20 minutes of vigorous activity at least three times a week

In addition to common recreational activities, such as walking, bicycling and dancing, the new guidelines promote routine activities such as mowing your lawn, gardening, washing the car, cleaning the house and climbing stairs.

An activity doesn't have to be condensed into one block of time in your busy schedule. The cumulative effect of physical activity throughout the day is what matters.

For example, taking a short bike ride in the morning, using the stairs instead of the elevator at work, and spending time working your flower beds in the afternoon can add up to be the equivalent of a single workout session at the gym. It all leads to better health.

However, not all types of daily activity count. The activity should be moderately intense, which could mean that your breathing quickens and you feel your heart beat a little faster. You can gauge this effort as being somewhere between 11 and 14 on the perceived exertion scale (see page 129).

That said, don't discount the benefits of vigorous exercise. The new guidelines are meant to complement — not replace — previous advice promoting high-intensity activities for people who are conditioned appropriately. More vigorous activity can bring greater health benefits. But the main point is that you take part in some type of physical activity for 30 to 60 minutes on most days of the week.

Perceived exertion scale

Exercise intensity reflects the amount of oxygen your body uses. The perceived exertion scale estimates exercise intensity. Perceived exertion is the total amount of effort and stress you feel during activity, including heart rate, breathing rate, perspiration and muscle fatigue.

The scale ranges from 6, representing your body at rest, to 20, representing maximal effort. Moderate activity ranges from 11 to 14. You can gauge your perceived effort while you exercise. For example, you adjust a brisk beach walk to what you perceive as about an 11 on the exertion scale in order to maintain a moderate pace.

6		14	
7	Very, very light	15	Hard
8		16	
9	Very light	17	Very hard
10		18	
11	Fairly light	19	Very, very hard
12		20	
13	Somewhat hard		

Copyright 1998 Gunnar Borg

Your perception of exercise intensity is more important than your absolute level of exertion. For example, brisk walking at 3 to 4 miles an hour may feel like light exercise to a physically fit person, but as strenuous exercise to someone who's not in shape. Both individuals will benefit from what they perceive as moderate exercise, although they'll walk at a different pace.

What kind of activity?

Physical fitness typically involves three components — aerobic activity to improve your heart and lung capacity (cardiovascular health), flexibility exercises to improve flexibility in your joints and muscles, and strengthening exercises to build and maintain bone and muscle mass.

Of these three components, aerobic activity has the greatest effect on blood pressure. But it's still important to practice all the components.

An activity is aerobic when it places added demands on your heart, lungs and muscles, increasing your body's ability to use oxygen. As a result, you can produce more energy and won't fatigue as quickly. It increases your endurance and stamina, so you can do the things you want to do.

How do I find the time to exercise?

Lack of time seems to be a common obstacle to exercise. But often, it's priorities rather than time that's the real issue. Being more physically active may require you to spend less time doing something else — perhaps a half-hour less spent watching television or surfing the Web.

- Walk for 10 minutes over your lunch hour, or get up a few minutes earlier in the morning and go for a short walk.
- Take regular activity breaks at work. Get up from your desk to stretch and walk around.
- Instead of looking for shortcuts from one location to another, look for opportunities to add an extra minute or two of walking.
- Schedule time with a friend to do physical activities together on a regular basis. This helps keep you motivated.

Cleaning house, playing golf or swimming laps all are aerobic activities if they require a fairly light to somewhat hard effort. Other common forms of aerobic activity include:

Walking. Walking appeals to many people because it doesn't require special athletic skills or instruction. It's convenient and inexpensive, and you can vary the route to keep it interesting. It's an activity that you can enjoy alone or with friends.

When walking, make sure you wear good shoes that give your feet support and traction. If you've been inactive and are out of shape, begin by walking at a very light pace for five to 10 minutes. Gradually increase the intensity and duration of your walks, as you can tolerate it. Your goal is to reach 30 to 60 minutes of exercise with each walk.

Jogging. Jogging is an excellent form of aerobic exercise because it provides a good workout for your heart, lungs and muscles in a relatively brief period of time. At the same time, jogging doesn't have to be strenuous to have a positive effect. You can go at your own pace. Like walking, jogging doesn't require a lot of equipment — just a good pair of shoes.

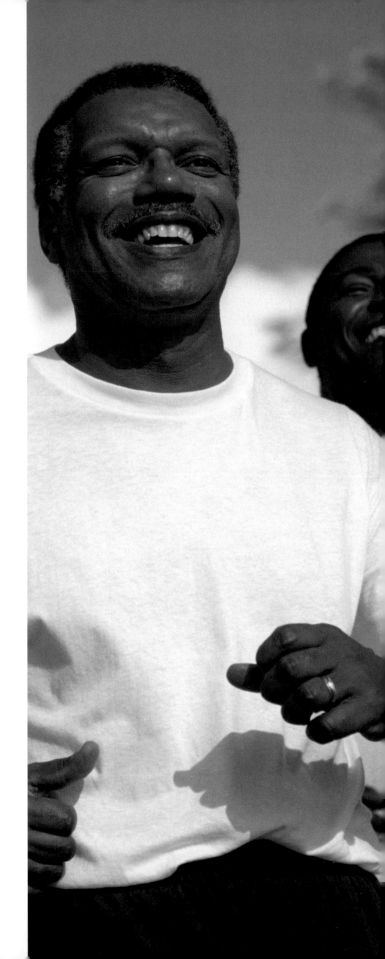

Be advised, however, that jogging requires some cardiovascular conditioning and muscle strengthening before you start. If you haven't been active for several months, begin by walking. When you're able to walk two miles (1.6 kilometers) in 30 minutes comfortably, you're ready to try alternating jogging with walking. Gradually increase the amount of time you spend jogging and decrease the amount of time you spend walking.

To minimize your risk of injury and muscle and joint discomfort, don't jog more than three or four times a week and try to jog on alternate days. If you have arthritis, this form of exercise can contribute to pain or discomfort in your knees, hips or ankles.

Bicycling. Like walking, bicycling is a good choice if you're just getting started on a regular exercise program. It's a low-impact activity that's great for people with joint problems such as arthritis. And bicycling offers a change of scenery with each session. Start slowly and build up your endurance to about 30 minutes or more three to six times a week.

You may be tempted to challenge yourself by setting the gears to make pedaling hard, producing a strain resembling that of a hard run. This gives you muscle fatigue but often doesn't work your heart and lungs effectively. Pedaling more rapidly at all times — 80 to 100 revolutions a minute — will help make your ride more aerobic.

If you're worried about traffic or don't care to chance the outdoors, a stationary bike is a good alternative. These machines can be upright or reclining (recumbent) and one type is not inherently better than the other — the choice is yours.

Stationary bikes give you mainly a lower body workout, but some have moving handlebars that increase the demands on your heart and lungs. If you have knee problems, adjust the resistance to a low setting, and keep your knees bent in the pedaling cycle.

Swimming and water exercise. Swimming is an excellent form of cardiovascular exercise because it conditions your heart and lungs as well as all the muscles in your body. It's also gentle to your joints. If you have arthritis or another joint disease, swimming is a good way to increase aerobic activity. Try to swim for 30 minutes several times each week.

Activity guide

Activity	Minutes required to burn 150 calories in 155-pound person*
Washing and waxing a car	45 to 60
Washing windows and floors	45 to 60
Playing volleyball	45
Playing touch football	30 to 45
Gardening	30 to 45
Wheeling self in wheelchair	30 to 40
Walking (20 minutes per mile)	35
Basketball (shooting baskets)	30
Bicycling (6 minutes per mile)	30
Dancing fast	30
Raking leaves	30
Water aerobics	30
Lawn mowing (push mower)	30
Walking (15 minutes per mile)	30
Swimming laps	20
Basketball (playing a game)	15 to 20
Jogging (12 minutes per mile)	20
Running (10 minutes per mile)	15
Shoveling snow	15
Stair climbing	15

*Equivalent to minutes required to burn 630 kilojoules in 70-kilogram person.

Adapted from National Institutes of Health. Clinical Guidelines on the Identification, Evaluation, and Treatment of Overweight and Obesity in Adults, 1998.

How do I know if I'm fit enough to exercise?

Fitness is an individual quality that's influenced by your age, sex, genetic makeup, eating habits, regular activity level and the presence of a chronic health condition. You'll know that you're fit if you can:

- Carry out daily tasks without getting overly tired and still have energy to enjoy leisurely pursuits
- Walk a mile or climb a few flights of stairs without becoming winded or feeling heaviness or fatigue in your legs
- Carry on a brief conversation using short sentences during moderate exercise such as brisk walking

If you're out of shape, you feel tired much of the time and fatigue quickly, you're unable to keep up with others your age, and you avoid certain activities because you know you'll soon tire.

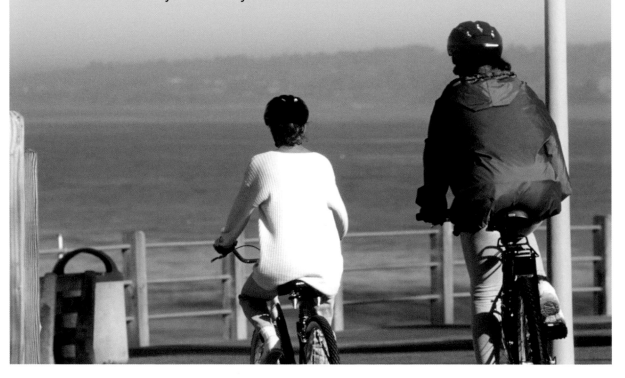

If lap swimming isn't your style, consider water aerobics or just walking in the pool. Because water provides about 12 times the resistance of air, walking in water about chest-high requires you to exert a certain amount of power to overcome the resistance. The water's buoyancy prevents falls and may aid circulation in people with blood flow problems in their lower extremities.

Exercise machines. Each of the six basic exercise machines offer specific fitness benefits to help you build aerobic capacity. In addition to the stationary bicycles mentioned previously, there are rowing machines, treadmills, stair climbers, cross-country machines and elliptical machines.

In general, you get what you pay for when you purchase an exercise machine. Look at the warranty — it's usually a sign of quality. Make sure the device is solidly built, with no exposed cables or chains, and that it operates smoothly. Avoid spring-operated components.

You can consult an expert at a local gym or fitness club to get their recommendations. They may allow you to try out different models.

How much activity?

No matter what activity you choose to do, your muscles and joints need time to get accustomed to different demands. If you've been inactive, start with five- or 10-minute periods of activity at a time and build up gradually in one-minute increments.

At first, try to exercise three times a week. Add more days after you've gotten used to exercise. Increasing the time gradually reduces the risk of injury and discomfort.

Your goal is to be as active as you can each day. At a minimum, aim to burn at least 150 calories daily doing aerobic activities. (See "Activity guide" on page 133.) For moderately intense activities, that equals about 30 minutes. Lighter activities require more time, and more vigorous activities less time.

The more you weigh, the less time it takes to burn calories — the less you weigh, the more time. However, if you use 30 minutes as your guide, you'll be close to getting the minimal amount of activity you need.

Remember, if it's difficult to carve 30 minutes out of your busy schedule, you can accumulate your activities in short intervals throughout the day. Go for a short walk before breakfast or during your lunch hour. Park your car farther away from work for a longer walk to the office door. Look for any opportunity to include more activity within your regular routine.

The six-step fitness plan below outlines how to start an activity program, how to add time or distance as your fitness improves, and how to add strength training to round out your overall fitness.

Basic fitness plan

Anyone can become more physically active. It's never too late to start, regardless of your age or weight or experience. But taking those first steps to being more active sometimes isn't as easy as it may seem.

Many people start to exercise but don't stick with it, often because they try to do too much too soon. An all-or-noth-ing mentality is a recipe for discouragement, not to mention possible injury. Tailor your expectations to your fitness level, health concerns, available time and motivation.

If you have a chronic health condition or you're at significant risk of cardio-vascular disease, special precautions before starting a program may apply. Check with your doctor first if you:

- Have regular blood pressure of 160/100 mm Hg or higher
- Have cardiovascular or lung disease, diabetes, arthritis, osteoporosis, kidney disease or any condition requiring medical care
- Have a family history of heart-related problems before age 55
- Are a man age 40 years or older or a woman age 50 or older
- Are unsure of your health status
- Have previously experienced chest discomfort, shortness of breath or dizziness following mild exertion

If you take medication, ask your doctor whether physical activity will change how the medication works. Drugs for diabetes and cardiovascular disease may cause dehydration, impaired balance and blurred vision. Some medications can also affect the way your body reacts to exercise.

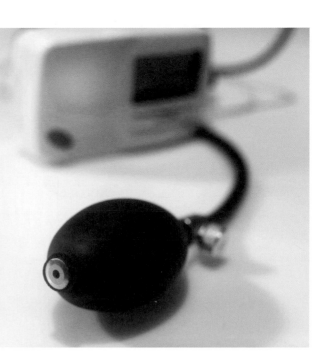

Exercise and your blood pressure

To get a true picture of your blood pressure level when you're home monitoring, measure it before you exercise instead of afterward. That's because your blood pressure may fall to a temporarily low level for a certain amount of time after exercising.

Set your goals

Goal setting is a way to meet your expectations and keep yourself motivated. To start your exercise program, try setting simple goals that are challenging but achievable in a reasonably short amount of time. It's easy to get frustrated and give up on goals that are too ambitious or that take too long to achieve.

Often, your overall goals (outcome goals) can be met through a series of smaller goals (performance goals) that build on each other.

For example, if you have high blood pressure, one of your outcome goals should be to reach a target blood pressure level set by you and your doctor. Another might be to lose weight. These outcome goals may be:

- I will lower my systolic blood pressure by 4 mm Hg and my diastolic pressure by 2 mm Hg within six months.
- I will lose 5 pounds (2.7 kilograms) in six months.

You can plan to achieve these outcomes with a series of performance goals. Here are some examples:

- I will avoid the elevator at work and use the stairs.
- I will be active at least 15 minutes every afternoon doing gardening, yardwork or housework.
- I will walk for 30 to 60 minutes three days a week.
- I will do strengthening exercises two days a week.
- I will stretch before and after all exercise.

Note that performance goals generally involve specific actions. Write all your goals down. Always be prepared to change or adjust them to suit your needs or to set new goals.

The success of performance goals can be measured by your mastery of each activity. Outcome goals help you focus on the desired result and keep you moving forward. People who can stay physically active for six months usually end up making it a habit.

Assemble your clothing and equipment

Your choice of exercise clothing depends on your activity and the weather or location where you exercise. Choose comfortable, nonrestrictive items that help you feel safe, supported and dry. It's better to underdress than to overdress because exercise generates body heat.

Today's active wear often uses high-tech performance fabrics that draw sweat away from the skin to the outer surface of the garment, where it can evaporate more quickly. These fabrics won't stop you from sweating, but they'll keep your skin drier.

Athletic footwear may be the single most important exercise item because for many activities, your feet take the biggest beating. Shoes should be the proper width, with cushioning or shock absorption, arch support, a degree of flexibility, and wiggle room for your toes.

Good walking shoes are stable from side to side and have a rocker sole design that encourages the foot to roll and push off the toes in a natural walking motion. It's fine to wear running shoes if your primary activity is walking, as long as your feet feel comfortable and supported.

If you primarily jog or run, steer clear of shoes designed for walking. Your feet sustain a more forceful impact when you run. The shoe should provide extra cushioning to protect bones and joints.

If you plan to bicycle, look for a helmet that's well ventilated and easy to use with snug straps. If you have trouble adjusting the helmet to fit your head, you're less likely to use it. A helmet should stay in place when pushed upward from the front and shouldn't tilt in any direction or slide. Try the helmet on before you buy it.

Make sure your bicycle is adjusted for your height and arm length. When you're seated with your foot on the pedal nearest the ground, your leg should be almost fully extended. You should be able to reach the handlebars and work the brakes and shift while keeping your eyes on the road.

Take time to stretch

Flexibility is the ability to move your joints through their full range of motion. You increase or maintain flexibility by regularly stretching your muscles, particularly before and after exercise. Stretching improves your coordination and posture, relieves stress and reduces your risk of injury.

Stretching for five to 10 minutes before an activity helps prepare your body for upcoming aerobic exercise. Be sure to warm up briefly before you stretch because stretching a cold muscle can strain the tissue. Simple stretches are illustrated on pages 141-142.

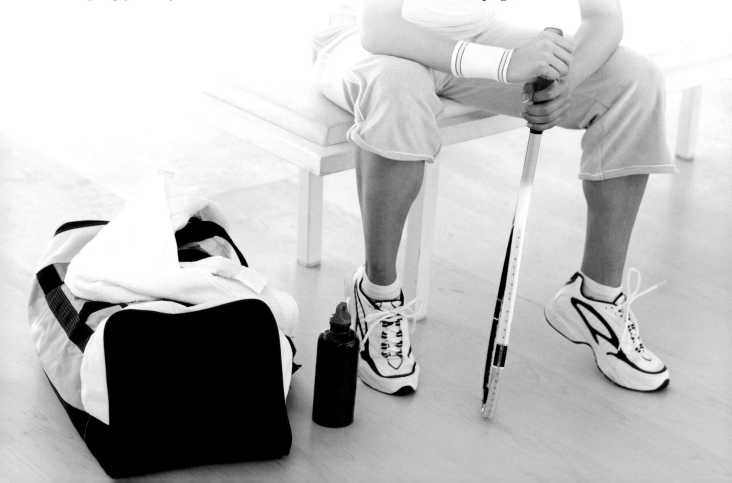

If you have time to stretch only once during a workout, stretch for five to 10 minutes after you exercise because, at this time, your muscles are loosened up and more receptive to stretching. This improves overall flexibility in your muscles and joints, and helps prevent muscle soreness.

Emphasize aerobic fitness

Spend at least 30 minutes doing an activity such as walking, jogging, biking and swimming. This will develop your aerobic capacity, which means your heart, lungs and blood vessels can efficiently transport large amounts of oxygen throughout your body. As a result, you can produce more energy and won't fatigue as quickly. You'll also burn more calories, control your appetite, increase your stamina and sleep better at night.

Depending on your level of fitness, aerobic activity should be fairly light to somewhat hard. If you've been inactive and are out of shape, begin with just three to five minutes at a very light pace. Then gradually increase your time by one to three minutes per session and increase your pace. Many people start a program with frenzied

zeal and then quit when their muscles and joints become sore or injured.

After you've been active for a while and you feel you're ready, gradually pick up the pace or increase the time you spend doing your activity by a few minutes each day. Instead of 30 minutes most days of the week, try aiming for 45 to 60 minutes.

When doing aerobic activities keep these suggestions in mind:

Mix your activities. Doing the same thing all of the time increases the chance that you'll become bored and lose interest in your program. Think of aerobic activities that are not the common forms, such as canoeing, ballroom dancing or water exercise. In addition, try to alternate among activities that emphasize lower and upper body fitness. Participating in more than one activity (cross-training) reduces your chance of overusing or straining a muscle or joint while underusing another.

Be flexible. On days when you're overly tired or not feeling well, don't force yourself to exercise. Be willing to take a short break from your program. And as soon as you're able, get back on track with an activity you enjoy.

Warm-up and cool-down stretches

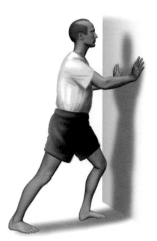

Calf stretch:

Stand an arm's length from the wall. Lean into the wall. Place one leg forward with knee bent. Keep other leg back with knee straight and heel down. Keeping back straight, move hips toward the wall until you feel a stretch. Hold for 30 seconds. Relax. Repeat with the other leg.

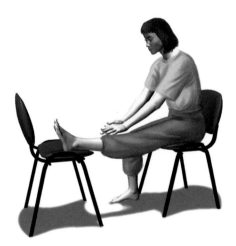

Hamstring stretch:

Sit securely on a low table or a chair with one leg propped on another chair. Without bending your knee, keep your back straight and lean forward until you feel a gentle pull at the back of your thigh. Hold the position for 30 seconds. Relax. Repeat with the other leg. (You can also do this exercise sitting on the floor with one leg out front and the other bent backward.)

Warm-up and cool-down stretches

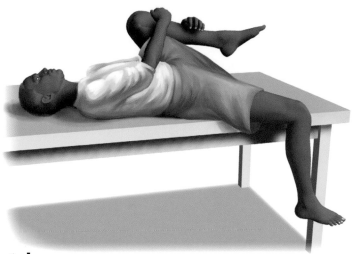

Upper thigh stretch:

Lie on a table or bed with one leg and hip as near the edge as possible and your lower leg hanging relaxed over the edge. Pull your other thigh and knee firmly toward your chest until your lower back flattens against the table. Hold for 30 seconds. Relax. Repeat with the other leg.

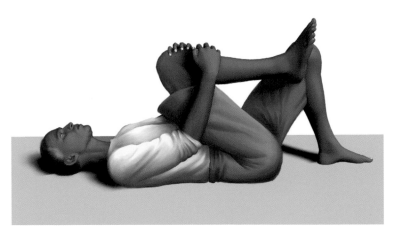

Lower back stretch:

Lie on a flat surface, such as the floor or a table, with your knees bent and feet flat on the surface. Grasp one knee and pull toward your shoulders. Stop when you feel a stretch in your lower back. Hold for 30 seconds. Relax. Repeat with the other leg.

Listen to your body. Start slowly and give your body a chance to get used to increased activity. Stretching is key to staying flexible and maintaining a range of motion in your muscles and joints. Muscle soreness after exercise is common, especially if it's new activity, but pain during exercise may send a different signal. Be aware of signs of overexertion or stress. (See "Avoiding injury" on pages 148-152.)

Build strength

At least twice a week, spend 20 to 30 minutes doing exercises that help build the strength and endurance of your muscles. Strength training is also called resistance training or weight training. This doesn't mean you'll bulk up. The increased lean muscle mass from these exercises simply provides you with a bigger "engine" to burn calories and control your weight.

Strength training is especially important as you get older because your muscle mass diminishes with age. Having greater muscle strength also makes aerobic activity easier. In addition, stronger muscles, tendons and ligaments around your joints help protect you from falls and fractures and reduce your risk of injury.

You build strength when your muscles push or pull against an opposing force, such as weight or gravity. The resistance can be achieved in many ways — moving or pushing against your own body weight, pulling on an elastic band or lifting weighted objects such as barbells and dumbbells.

The amount of weight or resistance you need to build muscle depends on your current strength. Choose a resistance that makes you feel as though you're working at a somewhat hard level. As you become stronger, you can increase the weight or resistance or the number of repetitions. See guidelines for strength training on page 146.

It's important to get instruction if you've never used strength training equipment before. You'll want to learn proper technique, safety precautions and different kinds of exercises to do with the equipment.

You can make your own weights by filling old socks with beans or pennies, or partially filling a half-gallon milk jug with water or sand. Or you can purchase used weights by the pound at some athletic equipment stores. A resistance band can help you work major muscle groups.

Simple strengthening exercises

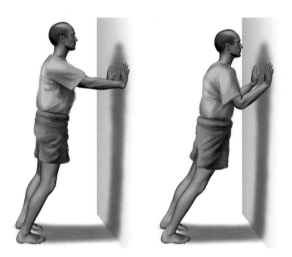

Wall push-up:

Face the wall and stand far enough away that you can place your palms on the wall with your elbows slightly bent. Slowly bend your elbows and lean toward the wall, supporting your weight with your arms. Straighten your arms and return to a standing position. This strengthens muscles in your arms and chest.

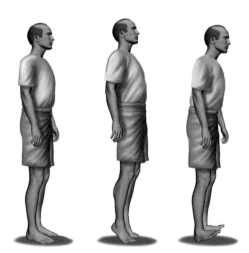

Toe and heel raise:

Standing, rise up so that your weight is on your toes. Then rock back and shift your weight to your heels, lifting your toes off the ground. This strengthens your calf and lower leg muscles to improve your balance.

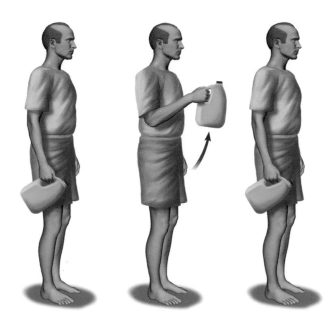

Arm curl:

Stand with your feet shoulder-width apart. For resistance, hold a partially filled half-gallon milk jug. Flex your elbow until your hand reaches shoulder height. Hold, then lower your arm slowly. This tones your biceps and helps in carrying and lifting. Remember to keep your wrist rigid while lifting — don't bend or curl your wrist.

Start with a weight you can lift comfortably eight times and build up to 12 repetitions. If you're a beginner, you may find that you're able to lift only 1 or 2 pounds in a set. That's OK. The weight should be heavy enough to tire your muscles but not cause pain.

If you start with too much resistance or too many repetitions, you may damage muscles and joints. Wait for your body to become accustomed to the exercise before gradually increasing intensity.

Find ways to stay motivated

Most people achieve a desirable level of fitness within three to nine months of starting their program. Your goal from then on is to maintain that level of physical fitness.

To keep yourself motivated:

Track your progress. Measure your progress with a written log or diary.

Guidelines for strength training

- Complete all movements slowly and with control. If you're unable to maintain good form and posture, decrease the weight or number of repetitions.
- If you have high blood pressure, consult your doctor before lifting heavy weights. The strain of lifting can cause a sharp increase in your blood pressure. This could possibly be dangerous if your high blood pressure is uncontrolled.
- Breathe normally and freely, exhaling as you lift a weight and inhaling as you lower it. Holding your breath during lifting can raise your blood pressure dramatically.
- Stop exercising immediately at the moment you feel any pain.
- Stretch your muscles before and after your workout. When stretching beforehand, warm up first by walking.
- It's normal to experience mild muscle soreness for a few days after starting strength training. Always allow at least one day in between strength training sessions so that your muscles can rest.

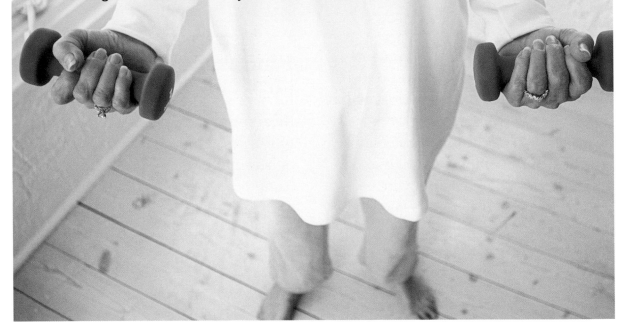

Seeing on paper how your fitness has improved can help keep you motivated to continue and do more.

Adapt your activities. As you become more fit, fine-tune the intensity and duration of your activities to better suit your interests and lifestyle.

Try new activities. Incorporating different and more challenging activities into your schedule will help keep your workouts enjoyable. Also look for ways to include family members in your physical activities.

Exercise and weight control

Regular physical activity, when combined with proper nutrition, does what hundreds of fad diets promise but never seem to deliver. It helps you lose weight and keep it off. Simply put, exercise burns calories. And when you burn more calories than you take in, you can reduce your body fat.

Here's how it works. Your body requires a certain amount of energy to maintain the functions you need to sustain life. When you exercise, your body works harder and needs more fuel (calories) to function. Even after you stop exercising, your body continues to burn calories at a modestly increased rate for a few hours. The more intensely you exercise, the more calories you burn.

According to the American College of Sports Medicine, people trying to lose weight should aim for 2 ½ hours of moderately intense exercise a week (or 30 minutes on five days of the week). Moderately intense exercise includes activities such as brisk walking, biking and swimming. If you can't reach that 2½ hour goal right away, that's OK. Work toward it.

Weight control combined with regular exercise reduces the risk of high blood pressure, even if you're already at a higher risk. Most studies have found that blood pressure is reduced relatively early — three weeks to three months — after starting an exercise program.

Although the generally recommended amount of exercise — 30 to 60 minutes most days of the week — can make positive changes, there's a caveat: When you stop exercising, blood pressure typically returns to its prior level.

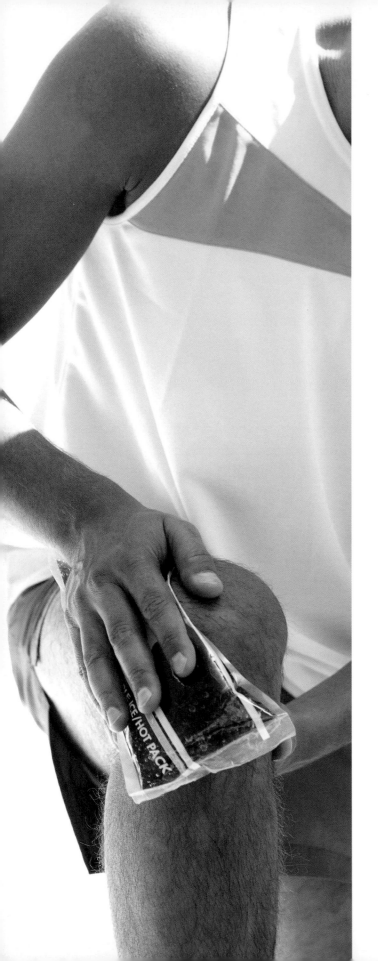

Physical activity helps you to not only lose weight but also to keep it off. So don't stop exercising just because you've lost a few pounds. Individuals who are at a healthy weight require just as much physical activity as do overweight people.

Avoiding injury

Everyone who's physically active is bound to feel some occasional soreness, stiffness or minor aches and pains. Muscle soreness that follows a day or two after exercise is normal, especially if you've been sedentary in the past or you're trying a new activity.

In fact, most injuries that occur during physical activity stem from the "terrible toos:" too much, too hard, too fast, too soon, too long. Pain during exercise can be a warning sign of impending injury. Gasping for breath and having sore joints are other signals that you need to slow down.

Just remember, if what you're doing hurts, then it's likely that you're over-doing it. It's time to consider reducing the intensity of the exercise or trying a different activity.

Another common cause of aches and pains is doing the same activities over and over without variation. This can lead to overuse injuries, caused by repeated stress on a particular part of your body.

You can reduce your risk of injury from exercise with the following tips:

Drink plenty of water. Water helps maintain your normal body temperature and cools working muscles. Exercise causes you to lose some of that water. To help replenish those fluids that you lose, drink water before, during and after activity.

Warm up and cool down. Stretching before a workout prepares your body for the upcoming activity. Stretching afterward helps improve your flexibility. Remember to warm up briefly before stretching cold muscles to avoid muscle strains.

Be active regularly. In general, the less fit you are, the greater your chance of getting injured. Avoid being a weekend warrior, when you reserve most of your activity for two days out of the week. Your risk of injury increases as you go back and forth between intense workouts and periods of inactivity.

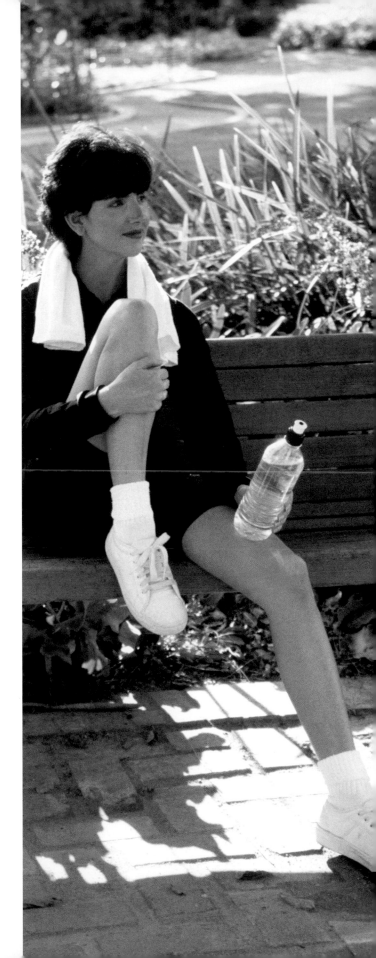

How can I exercise when I have painful arthritis in both of my knees?

For many people with pain problems, exercise can be beneficial. In the case of arthritis, proper exercise can help you better maintain joint mobility.

- Try water exercises. The buoyancy of water takes the weight off your joints. You can swim laps on your own or you might try a water aerobics class.
- Use a stationary or recumbent bicycle. This takes pressure off your knees.
- Consider joining a basic yoga or tai chi class to increase strength and flexibility in your joints.
- See a physical therapist who can offer recommendations on the best type of exercises for you and teach you how to do them properly to avoid injury and further pain.

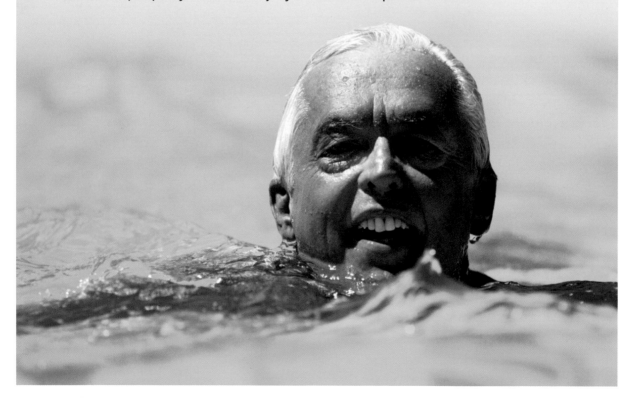

Follow the 10 percent rule. If you're planning to make your exercise more intense, limit these increases to about 10 percent. For example, if you swim laps for 30 minutes this week, plan to increase your workout to 33 minutes for the next week, and so on.

Avoid start-and-stop activities. A controlled, continuous form of activity, such as walking or cycling, generally produces less risk of a muscle pull or other injury than do activities in which you start and stop frequently, such as basketball or tennis.

Don't compete. Avoid the physical and emotional intensity that often accompanies competitive sports. A less stressful environment typically allows you to stay in control of your body and not overextend yourself.

Let food digest. Wait two to three hours after eating a large meal before being active. Digestion directs blood toward your digestive system and away from your heart.

Tailor your activity to the environment. When it's hot and humid weather, reduce your speed and distance. Or exercise early in the morning or late in the evening when it's cooler. Avoid activity near heavy traffic. Breathing carbon monoxide given off by automobiles reduces the oxygen supply to your heart.

Know the warning signs. Seek immediate care if you experience any of these signs and symptoms:
- Tightness in your chest
- Severe shortness of breath
- Chest pain or pain in your arms or jaw, often on the left side
- Fast, irregular heartbeats (palpitations)
- Dizziness, faintness or feeling sick to your stomach

What about illness?

If you're feeling tired or achy, should you exercise? The answer may depend on the illness you have. If you have a cold, moderate exercise won't make it worse or prolong it. If you have an infection accompanied by fever, exercising increases the risk of dehydration, dangerously high body temperature and even heart failure.

One common guideline for determining whether or not you should exercise is to do a "neck check." If your signs and symptoms are above the neck

— a stuffy or runny nose, sneezing or a sore throat — then moderate exercise is generally safe, although with caution. If you start feeling miserable, stop exercising.

Avoid intense activity if your signs and symptoms are below the neck. These include muscle aches, hacking cough, fever, extreme fatigue, vomiting, diarrhea, chills and swollen lymph glands.

Wrap-up

Key points to remember:
- Regular physical activity usually can reduce your blood pressure by 5 to 10 mm Hg.
- Exercising regularly is more important than the intensity of exercise.
- Get at least 30 minutes of moderately intense activity on most, if not all, days of the week.
- Aerobic activity has the greatest effect on blood pressure.
- If time for exercise is a problem, look for ways to include more activity in your daily routine.

Step 3

Avoid tobacco and limit alcohol

Despite substantial progress in the effort to curtail tobacco use, millions of people continue to smoke or use tobacco products. And odds are that you're part of the great majority of Americans who at least occasionally has an alcoholic drink.

Even if you're healthy, tobacco and alcohol can raise your blood pressure to an unhealthy level. Caffeine also may have an effect. If you have hypertension or you're at risk of it, you need to be especially alert to the effects that these substances can have on your blood pressure.

Tobacco and hypertension

Approximately one out of three people with high blood pressure smokes. Simply having hypertension puts you at increased risk of complications. But if you have high blood pressure and you smoke, you're two to three times more likely to develop cardiovascular disease than someone who doesn't smoke. And you're three to five times more likely to die of heart attack or heart failure. In addition, you're more than twice as likely to die of a stroke. These numbers are clear warnings about the dangers of smoking.

How smoking affects blood pressure

Tobacco contains a highly addictive drug called nicotine — the substance that makes it so difficult to stop smoking, even though you want to. It's also what causes your blood pressure to rise shortly after you take the first puff.

Like many other chemicals in tobacco smoke, nicotine is picked up by tiny blood vessels in your lungs and carried through your bloodstream. It takes only a few seconds for the drug to reach your brain. Your brain reacts to nicotine by signaling your adrenal glands to release epinephrine (adrenaline). This powerful hormone narrows your blood vessels, forcing your heart to pump harder under higher pressure.

The carbon monoxide in tobacco smoke replaces some of the oxygen carried in your blood. When your body doesn't get all of the oxygen it needs, your heart and lungs are required to work even harder. After smoking just two cigarettes, both your systolic and diastolic pressures increase an average of about 10 millimeters of mercury (mm Hg). Your blood pressure remains at this higher level for about 30 minutes after you finish smoking.

As the effects of smoking wear off, your blood pressure gradually decreases. However, if you smoke heavily, your blood pressure will remain at an elevated level throughout the day. If you smoke, regularly measure your blood pressure at home. Let your doctor know if your home readings are higher than those during your checkups.

Smoking has other damaging effects on your body. The chemicals absorbed from tobacco smoke affect the inner walls of your arteries, leaving them more susceptible to the buildup of fatty deposits (plaques) that narrow your arteries. Tobacco also triggers the release of hormones that cause your body to retain fluid. Both of these factors can lead to higher blood pressure.

Exposure to secondhand smoke also remains a serious health hazard. In terms of some of the negative effects on your blood vessels, even short exposure to secondhand smoke is believed to result in damage as serious as if the nonsmoker was actually the one who was doing the smoking.

Ex-smokers do win

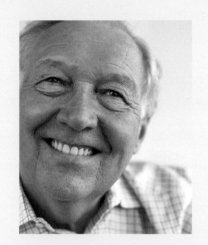

Many people continue to smoke because they believe they can't undo the damage already done to their bodies. Or they know too many other smokers who have tried to stop and failed. These assumptions are wrong.

Your body has an incredible capacity to repair itself. By the end of your first nonsmoking year, your risk of heart attack is reduced by 50 percent, and after five years it's almost the same as that for people who have never smoked. In addition, after 10 to 15 years your risk of getting lung cancer and other cancers associated with tobacco use is about half that of a smoker's risk.

It's true that most smokers aren't able to stop on their first attempt, particularly if they try to stop on their own. But stopping smoking is like learning anything else new. It often takes several attempts, and one bad experience shouldn't keep you from trying again. In fact, you can learn from previous attempts, increasing your chances for being successful in the future.

You can also enhance your chances for success by getting help from your doctor or by using a program that specializes in helping smokers stop. There also are more medications than ever before to assist you.

It's true that many people gain weight after stopping smoking. But the negative consequences of the added weight are usually more than offset by the positive health benefits of stopping smoking.

Each year in the United States, it's estimated that between 23,000 and 70,000 nonsmokers die of heart disease caused by secondhand smoke. If you have other risk factors for heart disease, it's imperative that you avoid secondhand smoke. Even if you don't have other risk factors, exposure to secondhand smoke is considered to be hazardous to your health.

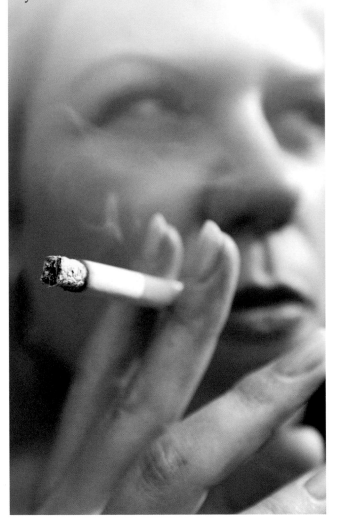

Why stopping is crucial

Not smoking may only slightly reduce your normal blood pressure. But it's still important to stop. Here's why:

First, smoking can interfere with some blood pressure medications, preventing them from working as well as they should, or sometimes from working at all. Second, having high blood pressure puts you at increased risk of a heart attack, heart failure and stroke because of the damage it can cause to your circulatory and neurological systems.

Smoking damages your arteries, producing the same cardiovascular risks as does high blood pressure. Therefore, when you combine high blood pressure with smoking, your odds for cardiovascular disease are much greater.

Breaking tobacco's grip

Some people can simply stop and never smoke again. Most people require several tries. But you *can* stop — many people have. And as you try, you can work with your doctor to stay in control of your blood pressure.

Becoming smoke-free is a result of planning and commitment, not luck.

Your stop plan should combine various strategies for:

- Coping with the symptoms of nicotine withdrawal
- Resisting urges to smoke
- Improving overall physical and emotional health
- Gaining social support and guidance, when necessary

Don't expect to find a ready-made stop plan for you to adopt as your own. No single plan works for everybody — there's no "right way" to stop smoking. Build a stop plan that you're comfortable with and that suits your needs.

Studies show that using or combining more than one strategy in your stop plan increases your chance of success. These strategies may include eating better, exercising, getting enough sleep and reducing stress.

Almost everyone experiences some symptoms of withdrawal when they stop smoking. For most smokers, the symptoms last for several weeks, becoming less intense and less frequent over time. Common symptoms include irritability, anxiety, nervousness and loss of concentration. Using one or more kinds of medication may help ease these symptoms.

Many weeks after your stop date, you may still have the desire to light up, particularly in familiar smoking situations such as after a meal. These urges and cravings are generally brief, but can be very strong and hard to resist.

Certain strategies in your stop plan may be to change behaviors or avoid situations that cause you to smoke. You may also identify alternative activities or distractions that help you resist the urges and cravings.

Most relapses take place within four weeks after stopping smoking. Often, the relapse occurs because of the overwhelming power of nicotine addiction and because the smoker hadn't developed a "fire escape" plan.

The following guidelines can increase your chances of success:

Do your homework. Read about the dangers of tobacco products and talk to people who have stopped or are trying to stop smoking. Consider your own smoking behaviors and plan for ways to prevent or avoid these situations. Identify your motivations for giving up cigarettes. This preparation helps you know what to expect when the day finally comes to stop smoking.

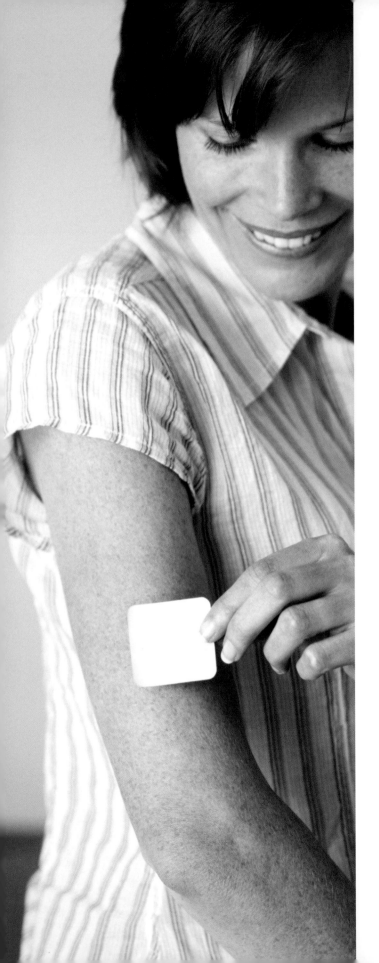

Set a stop day. Setting a firm date to stop smoking seems to work better than cutting back gradually. So carefully select a day when you throw your cigarettes away and no longer light up. Don't try to stop when you know your stress level will be high — although it's unlikely that you'll have a time when you're totally stress-free.

Consider medication and counseling help. The nicotine in tobacco products is highly addictive. Medications are available that can lessen the withdrawal symptoms and increase your comfort and sense of control (see sidebar on pages 160-161). Medications can't do all the work, but they can provide you with a better chance of success.

Research indicates that medication paired with counseling from a trained health care professional is even more effective. Ask your doctor about counseling services. In addition, many states and health organizations have telephone quit lines that provide advice and counseling. Some provide free nicotine patches or nicotine gum.

Tell others about your decision to stop. The support of family, friends and co-workers can help you reach your goal sooner. But many smokers

How do I change my smoking routine?

Before your stop day, try to separate smoking from everything else in your day-to-day life. Choose one location as a place to smoke, and don't smoke anywhere else.

- Buy cigarettes at a different location each time. Never return to the same place.
- Buy cigarettes in a single pack only. Never have more than one pack available at a time.
- When you smoke, do nothing else. Don't start associating smoking with any activity.
- Don't carry cigarettes with you. Keep your one pack in your designated smoking place.
- Don't carry a lighter or matches with you. Keep them (as well as ashtrays) with your one cigarette pack.

How do I cope with an urge to smoke?

- Remind yourself that the urge goes away in a few minutes.
- Keep your hands busy.
- Brush your teeth.
- Think about some aspect of smoking that's negative to you.
- Leave the situation for a few moments, if possible.
- Clear your mind and think about an enjoyable activity or relaxing place for a brief time.
- Call someone and talk about your feelings.

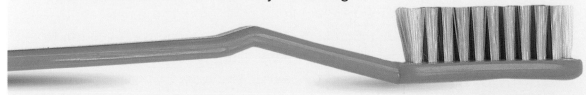

Medications to help you stop smoking

Most people use at least one medication when they try to stop smoking, but many find that a combination of medications is the most comfortable and effective approach. Use them according to your doctor's instructions or, in the case of over-the-counter (OTC) medications, according to instructions on the label.

Nicotine replacement products deliver small doses of nicotine to help relieve withdrawal symptoms but don't keep a smoker addicted to the substance. These products are considered temporary aids — usually for several weeks and at most several months. Consult your doctor about tapering off these medications.

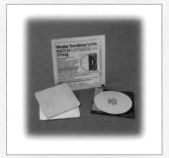

Nicotine patches. Similar to an adhesive bandage, a nicotine patch is placed on your skin and gradually releases nicotine into your body. It's an over-the-counter product and comes in different sizes — the larger the patch, the more nicotine delivered. To minimize skin irritation, rotate the site of the patch and apply an OTC cortisone cream.

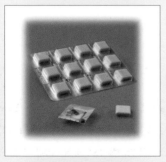

Nicotine gum. This OTC product is not intended to be chewed like normal gum. Bite into the nicotine gum a few times, then "park" it between your cheek and gum and leave it there. The lining of your mouth absorbs the nicotine that the gum releases. Two doses are available — 2 milligrams (mg) and 4 mg. Chew enough gum to relieve symptoms.

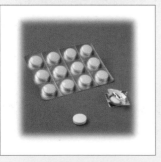

Nicotine lozenges. The nicotine lozenge was introduced as an OTC product in 2002. It looks like a hard candy and releases nicotine as it slowly dissolves in the mouth. Doses are available in 2-mg and 4-mg amounts — the 4-mg lozenge is used by heavier smokers.

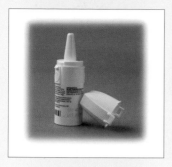

Nicotine nasal spray. You spray this product into your nose with a bottle dispenser. The nicotine is absorbed into your bloodstream through the lining of your nose, providing a quicker response to nicotine cravings than the other products provide. It's intended mainly for when you need immediate relief from withdrawal symptoms, and often used with nicotine patch therapy or with bupropion medication. The product is available only by prescription.

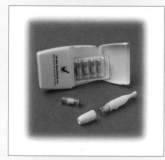

Nicotine inhaler. This device looks like a plastic cigarette that you put to your mouth and puff on, releasing a nicotine vapor into your mouth. Although it's called an inhaler, it doesn't deliver nicotine to the lungs. This product is available only by prescription and the dose is individualized. Using an inhaler also helps smokers who miss the hand-to-mouth ritual that's part of smoking a cigarette.

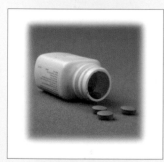

Non-nicotine medications. Bupropion (Zyban) is a non-addicting, non-nicotine medication approved by the Food and Drug Administration (FDA) as a stop-smoking aid. It's not clear exactly how the drug works. One theory is that bupropion stimulates dopamine, a brain chemical that causes a feel-good response similar to that produced by nicotine and other drugs of addiction. Bupropion is available only by prescription.

Varenicline (Chantix) is the most recent prescription drug approved by the FDA to stop smoking. This medication stimulates the same brain receptors that are usually activated by the nicotine in tobacco products. Chantix also blocks some of the pleasure you get from smoking, making smoking less rewarding.

choose to keep their plans a secret. That's because they don't want to look like a failure if they return to smoking.

Remember, it takes many people three or more tries before they can stop smoking for good. So there's no reason to feel like a failure just because your effort doesn't work out this time. Enlisting the support of at least one person can help you through a lapse.

Change your routine. Try to reduce the number of routine activities or situations that you identify with smoking before your stop day. That will make it easier to stop completely. For example, stop smoking inside your car or your house. This will help you become more comfortable being in those places without smoking.

You can also reduce the number of cigarettes you smoke before your stop day, but remember that your goal is to stop completely.

Take one day at a time. On your stop day, stop completely and each day following, focus your attention solely on remaining tobacco-free. Don't worry about tomorrow, next week or the "rest of your life." Just take it one day at a time, one urge at a time.

Avoid smoking situations. Stay away from situations in which you used to smoke. Leave the table immediately after meals if this was a time when you used to light up — go for a walk instead. If you always smoked while you talked on the telephone with friends, avoid long phone conversations or change the location where you talk. If you had a favorite smoking chair, don't sit in it anymore.

To some degree, you'll be able to recognize when an urge to smoke is about to hit you. Before it hits, start doing something that makes smoking inconvenient, such as making the bed, clearing the dinner table or washing the dishes. Smoking behavior is deeply ingrained and automatic — so you need to anticipate your reflex response to this urge and plan alternatives.

Time each urge. Check your watch when an urge to smoke hits. Most are short. Once you realize this, it may be easier to resist. Remind yourself, "I can make it another few minutes, and then the urge will pass."

Use medications along with other strategies to stop smoking. Remember that medications are just one part of an overall plan to change your behavior.

Alcohol and hypertension

There's a clear association between how much alcohol you drink and its effect on your blood pressure. So, if you drink alcohol, the best advice is to do so in moderation. Small amounts of alcohol don't seem to increase blood pressure and this is generally true even if you have high blood pressure.

Some evidence also suggests that moderate drinking may have certain cardiovascular benefits. For example, studies indicate that it can lower the risk of heart attack in middle-aged adults and may reduce the risk of blood clots, which can lead to stroke.

Moderate drinking also can boost the production of high-density lipoprotein (HDL or "good") cholesterol — the cholesterol that helps protect your arteries from the buildup of plaques. If

What's the best way to cut back on alcohol?

If you drink too much alcohol and you want to cut back, it's best to gradually reduce how much you drink over a period of one to two weeks.

People who drink heavily and suddenly stop consuming alcohol can develop severe high blood pressure that lasts for several days. One explanation is that when you suddenly remove alcohol from your bloodstream, your body releases abnormal amounts of the hormone epinephrine (adrenaline), which causes your blood pressure to rise sharply.

If you have high blood pressure and you drink more than a moderate amount of alcohol, talk with your doctor about the safest and most successful way to limit or avoid alcohol.

you didn't drink before, there's no reason to start now due to the potential problems with alcohol.

Unlike moderate consumption, excessive alcohol consumption is a problem for your cardiovascular system — along with many other negative health consequences. Drinking too much alcohol can increase your blood pressure and interfere with the function of your blood pressure medication. Heavy drinking may be responsible for about 8 percent of all cases of high blood pressure in the United States.

Moderate drinking — Less than you think?

Alcoholic drinks contain various amounts of the chemical ethanol (ethyl alcohol) — the more ethanol, the stronger the drink. For most men, moderate drinking is two drinks a day. Two drinks are equal to two 12-ounce (360-milliliter or mL) bottles of beer, two 5-ounce (150-mL) glasses of wine or two 1.5-ounce (45-mL) shot glasses of 80-proof liquor.

For women and small-framed men, moderate drinking is half that — one drink, or no more than half an ounce (15 mL) of ethanol daily. The amount is

less because women metabolize alcohol differently from men, and people with smaller builds have smaller volumes of blood, which results in higher concentrations of ethanol in their systems. For men and women age 65 and older, moderate drinking is one drink a day.

Remember that the effects of alcohol on your health are still being studied. Even moderate drinking may not be good for certain people. Be sure to consult your doctor about how alcohol consumption may affect your overall health and blood pressure.

How alcohol affects blood pressure

Exactly how excess alcohol — more than a moderate amount — increases blood pressure is unknown. One theory holds that alcohol consumption triggers the release of epinephrine (adrenaline) and other hormones that constrict your blood vessels or cause your kidneys to retain more sodium and water, raising blood pressure.

Excessive drinking is also associated with poor nutrition, which can deplete your levels of calcium and magnesium. A lack of these minerals in your body is associated with higher blood pressure. Your genes may also play a role in how alcohol affects blood pressure.

It's not only the amount of alcohol you consume but also when you consume it that can affect your blood pressure. A recent study suggests that people who drink alcohol outside of meals will have a significantly higher risk of hypertension, independent of the amount of alcohol they drink.

Regardless, it's clear that by reducing your alcohol consumption, you can reduce your blood pressure. Heavy drinkers who cut back to moderate levels can lower their systolic blood pressure by about 5 mm Hg and their diastolic pressure about 3 mm Hg.

Combining a healthy diet with reduced alcohol intake can produce an even larger reduction — a drop of about 10 mm Hg in systolic pressure and 7 mm Hg in diastolic pressure. One reason for this effect is that people who consume too much alcohol generally don't get adequate amounts of the minerals that help control blood pressure, such as potassium, calcium and magnesium.

People on blood pressure medication who limit alcohol consumption also tend to be more diligent about taking

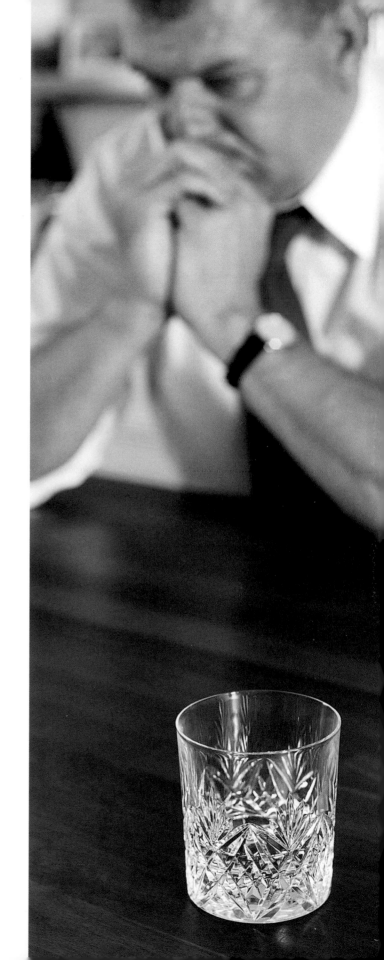

their medication. When influenced by alcohol, you may forget to take your pills or take them improperly.

Alcohol and medications

If you take any blood pressure medication, you need to pay careful attention to when or how you consume alcohol. Alcohol can interfere with the effectiveness of some medications and increase their side effects.

If you mix alcohol with a beta blocker, which relaxes your blood vessels and slows your heart rate, you may feel lightheaded or faint — especially if you're overheated or if you stand up suddenly.

You can experience the same symptoms if you drink alcohol close to the time you take an angiotensin-converting enzyme (ACE) inhibitor, which widens your blood vessels, or certain calcium channel blockers, which can slow your heart rate. If you do feel dizzy or faint, sit until the feeling passes. Drinking water also may help.

In general, any medication that causes drowsiness shouldn't be taken with alcohol. Read the medication label before you decide to consume alcohol.

And listen to your body. If you feel lightheaded or depressed after a drink or two, talk to your doctor about how much alcohol you can safely drink and when is the best time you can do it.

What about caffeine?

Caffeine is a mild stimulant found in coffee, tea, soft drinks and chocolate. It can fight fatigue, boost your concentration and lighten your mood. But if you use too much — something that's easy to do — caffeine can leave you jittery, cause your hands to tremble and possibly increase your blood pressure.

The amount of caffeine in two to three cups of coffee — 200 to 250 mg — has been shown to raise systolic pressure 3 to 14 mm Hg and diastolic pressure 4 to 13 mm Hg in people without high blood pressure.

Caffeine's influence on blood pressure remains an ongoing topic of debate. Some studies have found that people who consume caffeine regularly throughout the day will end up with higher average blood pressure than if

How do I reduce caffeine intake?

Caffeine can be habit-forming, so any attempts to stop or lessen the amount you normally consume can be challenging. An abrupt decrease in caffeine can cause withdrawal symptoms, such as headaches, fatigue, irritability and nervousness. These symptoms usually resolve after several days.

To adopt new caffeine habits, try these tips:

- Gradually reduce the amount of caffeine you consume. For example, drink one fewer can of soda or drink a smaller cup of coffee each day. This will help your body get used to the lower levels of caffeine and thereby lessen the effects of withdrawal.
- Replace caffeinated coffee, tea and soda with their decaffeinated counterparts. Most decaffeinated drinks look and taste the same.
- When preparing tea, brew for less time to cut down on its caffeine content. Or choose herbal teas, which don't contain this stimulant.
- Check the caffeine content in over-the-counter medications that you take. Pain relief or headache medications can contain from 65 mg to 130 mg of caffeine in one dose. Switch to caffeine-free versions, if possible.

they didn't consume any caffeine at all. However, other studies report that regular consumers of caffeine develop a tolerance to the stimulant. And after a while, at this regular level of consumption, caffeinated products don't have much effect on blood pressure.

Among people who don't consume caffeine on a regular basis or who consume greater amounts than they're used to, caffeine can cause a temporary but sharp increase in blood pressure. Exactly what causes this spike in blood pressure is uncertain.

Some researchers suggest that caffeine narrows your blood vessels by blocking the effects of adenosine (uh-DEN-o-sene), a hormone that helps keep the vessels widened. Caffeine may also stimulate the adrenal gland to release more cortisol and epinephrine.

As a general precaution, many doctors advise people with high blood pressure to limit daily caffeine intake to no more than two cups of coffee, four cups of tea or two to four cans of caffeinated soda to prevent any effects.

In addition, avoid caffeine right before activities that naturally increase your blood pressure, such as exercise or hard physical labor. Limiting caffeine is also good for your general health.

Wrap-up

Key points to remember:
- If you have high blood pressure and you smoke tobacco products, your risk of death from a heart attack, heart failure or stroke is much higher than if you don't smoke.
- It takes planning and commitment to stop smoking. Develop your own stop plan with coping skills, social support and strategies to deal with the symptoms of nicotine withdrawal.
- For many people, moderate alcohol use doesn't seem to affect blood pressure, but excessive alcohol use can have serious consequences for your cardiovascular system.
- Alcohol use may interfere with some high blood pressure medications or increase their side effects.
- Caffeine can cause a temporary but sharp rise in blood pressure, particularly among people who don't regularly consume caffeine. If you have high blood pressure, you may want to limit daily caffeine intake.

Step 4

Manage Stress

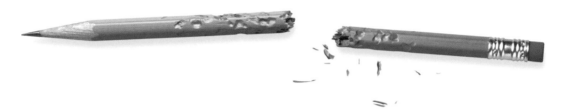

If you lead a stressful life, you'll have high blood pressure, right? This commonly held notion is not entirely true. There are many Type A individuals with normal blood pressure, just as there are laid-back individuals with high blood pressure.

It's true that when you're scared or under a tight deadline, your blood pressure may increase. As you relax, your blood pressure generally returns to normal. But chronic stress, in situations that aren't short-lived, may compound high blood pressure. Studies show that people who are characteristically impatient or hostile — traits commonly associated with stress — are more likely to develop hypertension.

If you have high blood pressure, reducing your stress may not lower your blood pressure completely. But less stress is important for other reasons:

Better long-term control. Even temporary increases in blood pressure caused by stress can make high blood pressure more difficult to manage. With less stress, you may have a better chance of staying in effective control.

More positive attitude. Stress can erode your commitment and motivation to control your high blood pressure. It's much easier to be physically active, eat a healthy diet, lose weight and limit alcohol when you're more relaxed and happy.

There are many ways to manage stress. You may want to experiment with different approaches and techniques until you have found stress relievers that fit your lifestyle and daily routine.

What is stress?

Think of stress as a spice. Too little spice results in a bland-tasting meal. Too much spice can muddle flavors or make the food inedible. When you use the correct amount, spice can provide a memorable eating experience.

Stress works in the same way on your health and well-being. You need some stress to keep your life interesting and challenging, but too much stress can overwhelm you. The issue is finding the right balance.

Positive and negative stress

Stress is a normal part of daily life. It's what you experience whenever you deal with demands that cause you to feel some degree of emotional or physical pressure and that challenge your ability to cope. It's important to know that stress is not the demands themselves (known as stressors) but rather how you respond to them.

Positive stress. Stress can provide feelings of excitement, opportunity and accomplishment. In these circumstances, you feel confident and motivated. Positive stress often drives athletes to perform well in competition. Other examples of positive stress may include working toward a college degree, getting married, starting a new job and experiencing childbirth.

Negative stress. Stress can make you feel out of control or overwhelmed. You may have trouble staying focused on the task at hand or feel isolated and "picked on" by others. Family relationships, financial affairs, work deadlines and poor health are common sources of negative stress. Major stress can be the sum result of many minor aggravations that have accumulated over time.

Physiologically your body tends to respond to any stressful challenge in the same way. How you perceive that challenge is what makes the stress positive or negative to you. Stress is therefore highly individualized. What may be stress for one person may not be stress for another. Some people generally cope well with difficult or tense situations, while others melt under the pressure. For a multitude of reasons, someone who dealt well with stress one week may have trouble coping with a similar kind of stress during the following week.

The stress response

Racing against a deadline, stuck in traffic, arguing with a spouse — these intense situations can make your body react as though you were facing a physical threat. The stress response, often referred to as the fight-or-flight response, switches your body into high gear. It provides you with the energy, speed, concentration and agility either to meet the challenge head-on (fight) or to get out of the way (flight).

This phenomenon can occur during any situation that's perceived — even falsely — as dangerous. In response to your perception of threat, a surge of hormones shifts your body into overdrive. Among the hormones are epinephrine (adrenaline) and cortisol, which cause your heart to beat faster and your blood pressure to increase.

? What are warning signs of stress?

Stress affects every body system and can cause many signs and symptoms, but some of the most common include:

- Overwhelming feelings of anger, frustration or anxiety
- Frequent headaches, backaches or colds
- Insomnia or other sleep disorders
- Increased use of alcohol or medications
- Feelings of grief, hopelessness or depression
- Diminished sense of humor
- Loss of interest in usual activities
- Periods of crying or other emotional outbursts
- Lack of attention to physical health and appearance

Just because you don't exhibit any of these symptoms does not mean you're not under stress. You may not recognize the symptoms, or you may be taking medications that mask them.

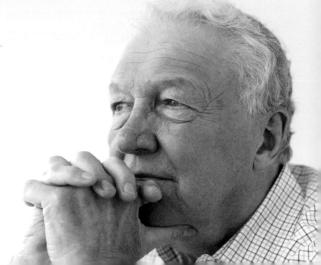

Other physical changes occur. Your breathing quickens, your blood sugar rises, and more blood and nutrients are sent to your brain and large muscles. Your body also releases chemicals that make your blood clot more easily. In a physical attack, this would help slow bleeding from a wound.

Your nervous system also springs into action. The pupils of your eyes dilate to enhance your vision. Your facial muscles tense up to make you look more intimidating. You perspire to cool your body.

Your mind has ways of letting you know when it's under too much stress. You may become easily discouraged, irritable, cynical, emotional or even reclusive. All of these feelings affect how you think and act. However, the changes can sometimes be easy to miss because they develop gradually and with little warning.

Physical signs and symptoms of stress aren't as easy to ignore. They may include headache, stomach upset, insomnia, fatigue and frequent illness. You may find yourself reverting to nervous habits, such as biting your nails or smoking. You might turn to alcohol or drugs.

Stress and blood pressure

The hormones epinephrine and cortisol released during periods of high stress increase blood pressure by narrowing your blood vessels and increasing your heart rate. The increase in blood pressure caused by stress varies, depending on how intense your stressor is and on how your body copes with the challenge. In some people, stress causes only a slight increase in blood pressure. In others, stress can produce extreme jumps in blood pressure.

Nevertheless, the effects of stress on your body are usually only temporary. However, if you regularly experience high levels of stress, the increases in blood pressure can over time start to damage your arteries, heart, brain, kidneys and eyes. This cumulative effect of stress often goes unrecognized until the condition manifests itself as persistent high blood pressure.

Strategies for relieving stress

It's one thing to be aware of stress in your daily life. And it's another thing to do something about it.

Stress and your health

Stress is thought to play a role in several medical conditions. When your heart rate increases, you become at greater risk of chest pain (angina) and irregularities in your heart rhythm (arrhythmia). Stress-related surges in your heart rate and blood pressure can also trigger a heart attack or damage your heart muscle or coronary arteries. The blood-clotting protein fibrin released when you're under stress also puts you at increased risk of blood clots.

The hormone cortisol is released during stress, and it may suppress your immune system. There's evidence that this suppression may make you more susceptible to infectious diseases, including upper respiratory viral infections such as cold or flu.

Stress can also trigger headaches and may worsen asthma and intestinal problems. It may also interfere with wound healing.

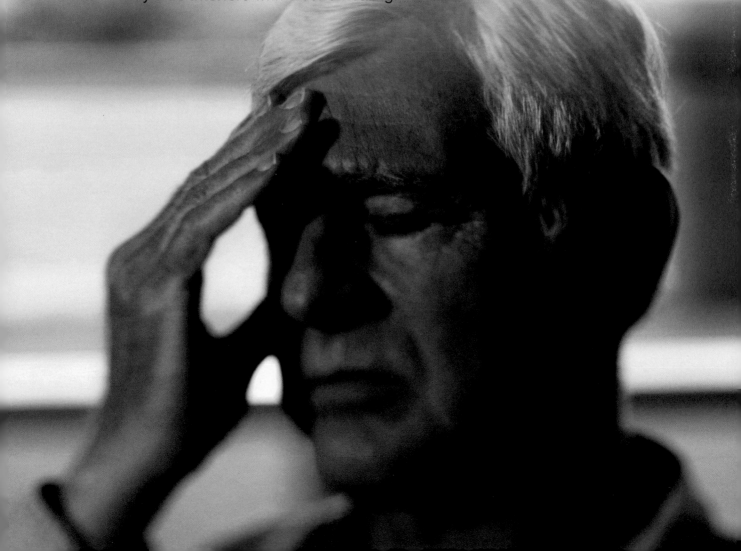

Stress becomes a problem when the demands placed on you threaten to overcome or exceed your ability to cope. To stay on track through stressful times, try this four-step strategy:

Take stock of your stress. Consider the particular circumstances that may have caused a situation when you're feeling overwhelmed or upset. Write these factors down in a list. Keep in mind that stress can be caused by external factors — for example, family relations or unpredictable events — as well as by internal factors — such as negative attitudes or unrealistic expectations.

Examine your stressors. Try to identify the problem at its root. Then ask yourself, "How can I change this situation?" or "How can I improve my ability to cope with stress?" Once you know what's at the root of your stress, you can take steps to deal with it.

Evaluate your needs and responsibilities. Assess the activities in your daily life and prioritize which ones are most important to you. Determine the tasks that you can most easily adapt or change. If you feel overcommitted, can you delegate some of the tasks to others or ask them for help? Can you say no to new responsibilities?

Learn to relax. Develop coping strategies that help you relax when you feel yourself becoming stressed. Proven stress-reduction strategies include exercise, relaxed breathing and muscle relaxation techniques, as well as simply learning to laugh.

Following are additional guidelines to accomplish stress relief.

Changing your lifestyle

Making simple changes in your daily routine can often lessen your stress level. These changes include:

Get organized. Prepare a written schedule of your weekly activities, highlighting priority tasks. This exercise will help reduce time conflicts, missed appointments and last-minute deadlines. Schedule important tasks — especially those that seem most stressful — at the time of day when you're feeling your best.

Simplify your schedule. Try to adopt a more relaxed pace. Assess your time commitments, and don't feel guilty or obligated if you say no to job requests or social invitations that you know you can't handle. Look to others for help or delegate responsibilities.

Relieve work-related stress. Job frustration can be a major source of stress. To relieve the worry and disappointment, look for ways to upgrade your job performance. Take time to do high-quality work but don't strive for perfection. Show respect for others and a willingness to resolve conflicts with co-workers. Identify skills you'll need for your long-term career goals and create a plan for developing those skills.

Build a financial cushion. Try to put aside a portion of every paycheck into a savings account or low-risk investment. Having reserve funds in the bank is one way to cope with unexpected financial stress such as the loss of a job, a salary cut or a large, unplanned-for expense. Even if an emergency use for the money never arrives, knowing that you have a financial cushion can reduce anxiety.

 ## How do I stay in control of stressful situations?

When you're trying to manage stress, consider one of the four A's when you're looking for a solution:

Avoid. A lot of needless stress can simply be avoided. Don't like traffic jams? Leave for work early. Hate waiting in line at the cafeteria? Pack a lunch. Put physical distance between you and a person who bothers you.

Alter. Try to change your situation, so things will have a chance to work better in the future. Respectfully ask others to change their behavior and be willing to do the same. Manage your time better. Take some risks.

Adapt. Changing your standards or expectations is one of the best ways to deal with stress. Look at your situation from a new perspective. Think more about the positives in life and less about the negatives. Focus on the big picture.

Accept. If you have no choice but to accept things as they are, try to forgive and smile. Talk to a friend. Learn from your mistakes.

Exercise. In addition to helping control your blood pressure and reduce your weight, exercise also alleviates daily tensions and reduces the symptoms of mild depression and anxiety. The energy and optimism that can result from exercise helps you stay calm and think clearly. Exercise 30 to 60 minutes on most days of the week.

Eat well. Stress and overeating go hand in hand. Many people turn to high-calorie, high-fat comfort food

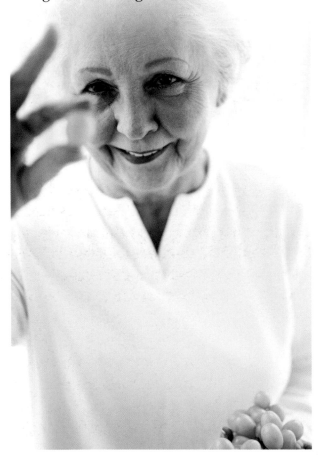

when they're dealing with a difficult problem or are at a weak emotional point. If the urge strikes, try to distract yourself by calling a friend or going for a walk. When your mind is occupied, the urge can quickly go away.

A healthy approach to eating includes a wide variety of foods that are good tasting and simple to prepare. This diet emphasizes vegetables, fruits and whole grains, which are packed with nutrition but are low in calories for their bulk — so they fill you up but not out. These foods contain antioxidants, dietary fiber and other disease-fighting substances that help keep your body systems in good working order.

Get plenty of sleep. When you're refreshed from a good night's sleep, you're better able to tackle the next day's problems. Going to bed and awakening at consistent times each day can help you sleep better. Slow the pace of your evening activities to establish a calming environment. A bedtime ritual, such as reading or listening to music, can aid in falling asleep.

Straighten up. Observe your posture and physical bearing when you feel overly stressed. You may find that you slump your shoulders, your breathing becomes shallow and you're less active. Stress may cause you to neglect your appearance and avoid people.

Good posture helps relieve aches and pains by placing minimal strain on your muscles and allowing you to move efficiently. Stand with your weight on both feet, shoulders back and stomach muscles tight. Keep your back well supported when you're seated. Stick to your regular routines and take time for good grooming.

Take occasional breaks. Take opportunities to stretch, walk and relax during your regular day. Use brief vacations, even if they're just for a day or the weekend, to leave stressful problems behind. Pursue hobbies and recreational activities that you enjoy. Quality leisure time reduces stress and improves your outlook on life.

Maintain social relationships. Friends and family can provide a valuable release valve when you need to vent your emotions. They can also give you encouragement and helpful advice. However, try to avoid confiding with individuals who tend to be negative about everything and who foster bad feelings. Try to surround yourself with people who will support you.

Thinking positively

Studies indicate that an optimistic attitude helps you to cope better with stressful situations, likely reducing the effects that stress has on your body. On the other hand, a pessimistic outlook can make it much harder to deal with even minor aggravations.

Monitor self-talk. The endless stream of thoughts that run through your head can be positive or negative. You can reduce stress by learning how to halt negative thoughts and practice positive thinking. For example, instead of telling yourself "I should never make a mistake because I'll look foolish," try thinking "Everyone makes mistakes, and I will be more careful next time." This approach can make your outlook more realistic and self-affirming.

Manage your anger. Everyday frustrations can cause your temper to flare. But if your blood boils after even minor irritations or you're constantly seething, you may need to work at getting your anger under control. Anger itself isn't bad and, when expressed appropriately, can be healthy. But anger that's out of control is destructive, leading to problems in your relationships, health and enjoyment of life.

How can you control anger? Think carefully before saying something you'll later regret. Take a time out — count to 10 before reacting or leave the situation entirely if you can. Find ways to calm and soothe yourself. Express your anger as soon as possible in a controlled manner so that you aren't left stewing. And don't hold a grudge.

Look for humor. Laughter is a natural high — it doesn't just lighten your load mentally, it actually induces physical reactions in your body. When you laugh, your heart, lungs and muscles are stimulated. Just 20 seconds of laughter produces an oxygen exchange that equals about three minutes of aerobic exercise. Laughter also releases chemicals in your brain called endorphins that ease pain and enhance a feeling of well-being. If you use humor to deal with setbacks positively, you're less likely to feel sorry for yourself.

Schedule worry time. Setting aside a time for problem solving can prevent your worries from building up inside you. Devote time each day to work on solutions to problems that are causing stress and assess your progress in solving them. If a worry crops up outside of worry time, write it down and worry about it later.

Learning to relax

Not all stress is avoidable. There are certain events in life that you can't prevent, such as getting stuck in an unexpected traffic jam. But you can reduce the emotional and physical toll these events can take on you.

When you're feeling stressed, take a moment to relax your body and clear your head. The following exercises are designed to help you achieve this. However, keep in mind that relaxation doesn't happen automatically. For you to develop this skill, you need to practice it daily. If you're not successful, consult a qualified professional.

Relaxed breathing. Stress typically causes rapid, shallow breathing from your chest, which sustains other aspects of the stress reaction, such as rapid heart rate and perspiration. You breathe correctly when you're breathe deeply from your diaphragm, and your abdomen — not your chest — moves with each breath.

Deep, slow breathing from your diaphragm is more relaxing. It also exchanges more carbon dioxide for oxygen to give you more energy. This kind of breathing acts on centers in your brain that lower blood pressure. If you're able to control shallow breathing and to relax, the effects of acute stress will decrease (see page 180).

A medical device called Resperate is designed to help lower blood pressure with deep breathing. The device includes a respiration sensor, headphones and a small unit that looks like a portable CD player. Resperate analyzes your breathing pattern and then creates two distinct melodic tones to guide your inhalation and exhalation. If you're synchronized to the melody, you can slow your breathing to fewer than 10 breaths a minute.

To achieve a lasting reduction in systolic pressure, you'll need to use Resperate for about 15 minutes several days a week. If you stop doing the breathing exercises, your systolic pressure will rise again.

Muscle tension exercises. Mounting tension and stress can cause your muscles to tighten, especially in your shoulders. To relieve the tightness, roll your shoulders, raising them toward your ears. Then relax your shoulders.

To reduce neck tension, gently move your head clockwise in a circle, then counterclockwise. To relieve tension in your back and torso, reach toward the ceiling and do side bends. For foot and leg tension, draw circles in the air with your feet while flexing your toes.

Progressive muscle relaxation can help reduce tension, anxiety and stress related to conditions such as high blood pressure and depression. Beginning with your feet and working up through your body to your head and neck, tense each muscle group for at least five seconds and then relax the muscles for up to 30 seconds. Repeat before moving to the next muscle group.

Guided imagery. Also known as visualization, this method of relaxation relies on memories, dreams and fantasies to see with your "mind's eye." You experience a peaceful setting with all of your senses, as if you were actually there, imagining the sounds, scents, colors and tactile sensations. The messages your brain receives from this imagery help your body to relax. Research has shown that these mental images produce physiological, biochemical and immunological changes in the body that impact health.

Meditation. In meditation, you focus attention on your breathing, or on

Taking a breather

Here's an exercise to help you practice relaxed breathing.

1. Wear comfortable clothes that are loose around your waist. You may lie on your back or sit in a chair, as you prefer.
2. Lie with your feet slightly apart, with one hand resting on your abdomen and the other hand on your chest. If you're sitting, place your feet flat on the floor, relax your shoulders and place your hands in your lap or at your side.
3. Inhale through your nose, if you can, because this filters and warms the air. Exhale through your mouth.
4. Concentrate on your breathing for a few minutes, then gently exhale most of the air in your lungs.
5. Inhale while slowly counting to four, about one second per count. As you inhale, slightly raise your abdomen about an inch (2.5 centimeters). You should be able to feel the movement with your hand.
6. As you breathe in, imagine the air flowing to all parts of your body, supplying you with cleansing, energizing oxygen.
7. Pause for a second with the air in your lungs. Then slowly exhale, counting to four. You'll feel your abdomen slowly fall as your diaphragm relaxes. Imagine the tension flowing out of you.
8. Pause for a moment. Then repeat this exercise for one to two minutes, until you feel better. If you experience lightheadedness, shorten the length or depth of your breathing.

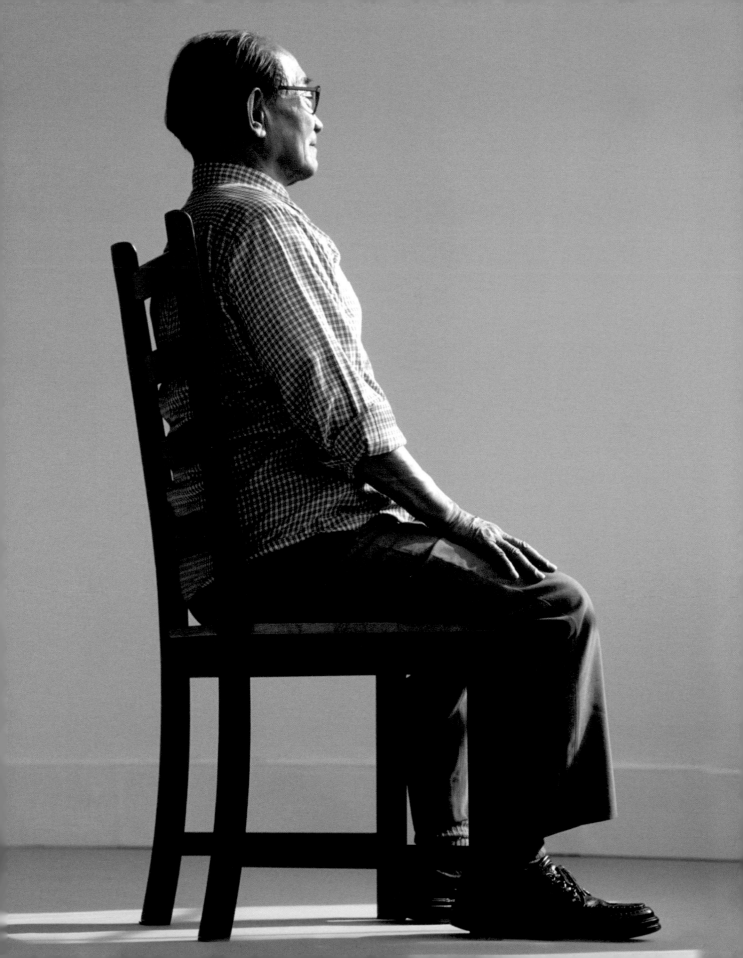

repeating a word, phrase or sound in order to clear your mind of distracting thoughts. Most types of meditation require four elements: a quiet place, specific posture, focused attention, and open attitude that allows distractions to come and go without suppressing them. Rather, you gently bring your attention back to the focus.

Meditation is believed to lead to a state of physical relaxation and psychological balance. It's also been shown to affect your body's stress reaction. One study found that people with high blood pressure who practiced meditation were able to reduce their blood pressure and lower their heart rate.

Professional help

Sometimes, life's problems pile up and become more than you can deal with on your own. When you feel over-whelmed by stress, consider getting help from your doctor or a qualified behavioral counselor. Some people believe that seeking outside help is a sign of weakness. Nothing could be further from the truth. It takes strength of character to admit you need help.

Learning how to control stress won't guarantee you'll have a normal blood pressure, let alone a relaxed life and good health. Unexpected problems will still occur. But having the tools to cope with stress can make those problems easier to overcome — and your blood pressure easier to control.

Wrap-up

Key points to remember:
- Stress can increase your blood pressure temporarily and complicate existing high blood pressure.
- Over time, the physical effects of stress can be damaging to your health and well-being.
- Although reducing stress may not completely lower your blood pressure, it can make your blood pressure easier to control.
- Lifestyle changes, relaxation techniques and professional help can help you avoid or better manage stress and reduce health risks.

Step 5

Get the right medication

 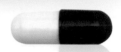

Making changes in your lifestyle is a fundamental way to control blood pressure, for example, by adjusting your diet, getting more exercise and stopping smoking. These measures are considered a first line of therapy for high blood pressure and are typically started early in any treatment program. Often, lifestyle changes simply aren't enough. To reach a desirable blood pressure level, you may also need the help of medication.

In case of stage 2 high blood pressure, medication is often required to reduce the pressure further and more rapidly than any lifestyle change could ever accomplish. If other conditions accompany your high blood pressure, medications may also be necessary.

Blood pressure medications, known as antihypertensives, are a major success story in modern medicine. They're quite effective, and most people aren't bothered by their side effects. These drugs can allow you to live normally with controlled blood pressure but also provide benefits by reducing your risk of other health concerns.

There are several classes of blood pressure medication, and each class affects blood pressure in a different fashion. If one drug is prescribed but doesn't lower your blood pressure to a safe level, your doctor may substitute a different drug or add another medication to the prescription you already have. Two or more low-dose drugs in combination may be able to lower blood pressure as well as or better than one drug alone can at full dose. In addition, using lower doses in drug combinations may produce fewer side effects.

Finding the right medication — or combination of medications — may take time. This is especially true if you have a condition when a lower target blood pressure level is required. Other factors to consider when deciding on the best medication include your age and overall health, other medications you are taking, how often you take the drugs,

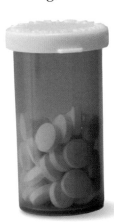

how you feel while taking them, and the total cost of medication. What's important is that you're working with your doctor to develop a treatment plan that's tolerable, cost-effective and personalized.

Many options

The major classes of medication used to control high blood pressure include:

- Diuretics
- Beta blockers
- Angiotensin-converting enzyme (ACE) inhibitors
- Angiotensin II receptor blockers (ARBs)
- Renin inhibitor
- Calcium channel blockers (calcium antagonists)
- Alpha blockers
- Alpha-beta blockers
- Central-acting agents
- Direct vasodilators

The following sections list drug names alphabetically with the generic name first. If you have questions about a medication, talk with your doctor.

Diuretics

Diuretics were first introduced in the 1950s, and are still some of the most commonly used medications to lower blood pressure. Diuretics have two major advantages over some of the other high blood pressure drugs. First, diuretics are the least expensive of all the blood pressure drugs. Second, they've repeatedly proved their effectiveness over the years, for example, in the Antihypertensive and Lipid-Lowering Treatment to Prevent Heart Attack Trial (ALLHAT), published in late 2002. ALLHAT researchers found that among about 33,000 people age 55 and older, treatment programs based on diuretics were more effective than those for ACE inhibitors or calcium channel blockers in controlling high blood pressure and preventing cardiovascular disease.

Commonly referred to as water pills, diuretics reduce the volume of fluid in your body. They signal your kidneys to excrete more sodium in your urine than they would normally. The sodium takes with it water from your blood. This effect means there's a smaller volume of blood pushing through your arteries and, consequently, less pressure on your artery walls.

Diuretics are often the first drug of choice for people with stage 1 high blood pressure. They're highly effective in blacks and older adults, who more frequently are sodium sensitive. In addition, they're commonly used in combination with other medications.

If you take a diuretic, it's important that you also limit sodium and get enough potassium in your diet. This will help the drug work more effectively and with fewer side effects.

Types of diuretics

There are three types of diuretics. Each works by affecting the nephrons, the filtering units of your kidneys.

Thiazides. Listed below are thiazide and thiazide-like diuretics:
- Bendroflumethiazide (Naturetin)
- Chlorothiazide (Diuril)
- Chlorthalidone (Hygroton, Thalitone)
- Hydrochlorothiazide (HydroDiuril, Microzide)
- Indapamide (Lozol)
- Methyclothiazide (Aquatensen, Enduron)
- Metolazone (Mykrox, Zaroxolyn)
- Polythiazide (Renese)

In addition to controlling high blood pressure, thiazide diuretics provide other potential benefits. They've been shown to reduce the risk of stroke, heart attack and heart failure in older adults. They also reduce the amount of calcium in your urine, so less calcium is available for kidney stone formation.

Less calcium in your urine means more of this mineral remains in your blood, helping to reduce your risk of osteoporosis and hip fracture.

Loop. These diuretics are more powerful than thiazides, removing a greater amount of sodium from your kidneys. They may also remove more calcium, although proper monitoring can prevent complications. Your doctor may recommend a loop diuretic if thiazides aren't effective, particularly if you have chronic kidney disease, or if you have other conditions that cause your body to retain fluid.

Loop diuretics include:
- Bumetanide (Bumex)
- Ethacrynic acid (Edecrin)
- Furosemide (Lasix)
- Torsemide (Demadex)

Potassium-sparing. In addition to removing sodium from your blood, thiazide and loop diuretics remove potassium. Potassium-sparing diuretics help your body retain needed potassium. This type of drug is used mainly in combination with other diuretics because they aren't as powerful as the thiazide or loop varieties. When taken with other drugs, the potassium-sparing diuretic spironolactone also reduces deaths from heart failure and is particularly effective with resistant high blood pressure. Eplerenone is an improved version of spironolactone that appears to have fewer side effects.

Potassium-sparing diuretics include:
- Amiloride (Midamor)
- Eplerenone (Inspra)
- Spironolactone (Aldactone)
- Triamterene (Dyrenium)

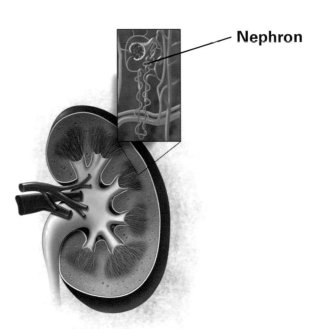
Nephron

Diuretics and your kidneys

Nephrons are the filtering units of your kidneys — tiny bundles of intertwining blood vessels and tubules. Each organ is packed with about 1 million of them. The different types of diuretics act on different parts of the nephron.

Side effects and cautions

The most common side effect of diuretics is increased urination. Thiazide and loop diuretics can also cause low potassium levels. That's why the two are often used with a potassium-sparing diuretic, ACE inhibitor or ARB.

Thiazide diuretics may cause dizziness in older adults upon standing. They can also cause impotence in some men, although this is uncommon. In addition, thiazides in high doses can slightly increase your blood sugar and cholesterol levels. They also increase the level of uric acid in your blood, leading, in rare cases, to the development of gout, a joint disorder.

Another rare condition, known as hyponatremia, involves low levels of sodium in your blood. It often occurs in older adults who are taking thiazide diuretics and who drink too much water. Hyponatremia causes headache and confusion, and can lead to coma.

Loop diuretics can sometimes lead to dehydration. Potassium-sparing diuretics may raise your potassium level too much. If you have impaired kidney function, you shouldn't take a potassium-sparing diuretic.

Beta blockers

Beta blockers lower blood pressure by blocking many of the effects of the hormone epinephrine (ep-ih-NEF-rin), also known as adrenaline (uh-DREN-uh-lin). The action of a beta blocker makes your heart beat more slowly and less forcefully, thus helping to lower your blood pressure.

These drugs also slow your kidneys' release of the enzyme renin. Renin is involved in the production of a substance called angiotensin (an-je-o-TEN-sin) II, which narrows your blood vessels and increases your blood pressure.

Like diuretics, beta blockers have been used for many years and lower blood pressure in most people who try them. Beta blockers alone may not be the first choice for cases of uncomplicated hypertension — a better choice may be in combination or with another drug option — but they're especially helpful if high blood pressure is accompanied by cardiovascular conditions such as chest pain (angina), irregular heart rhythm (arrhythmia), heart failure or previous heart attack. They help control these conditions and reduce your risk of a second heart attack.

Beta blockers work especially well in older adults who have heart disease. However, blacks don't respond as well as whites do when taking most types of beta blockers as a single drug.

These drugs were originally developed to treat coronary artery disease and were later approved for the treatment of high blood pressure after studies found they could lower blood pressure. They may also be used to treat glaucoma, migraines, anxiety, hyperthyroidism and some tremors.

Types of beta blockers

Beta blockers can affect your heart (cardioselective) or both your heart and blood vessels (noncardioselective). The cardioselective drugs generally produce fewer side effects. Beta blockers used to treat hypertension include:
- Acebutolol (Sectral)
- Atenolol (Tenormin)
- Betaxolol (Kerlone)
- Bisoprolol (Zebeta)
- Carteolol (Cartrol)
- Metoprolol (Lopressor, Toprol-XL)
- Nadolol (Corgard)
- Penbutolol (Levatol)
- Pindolol (Visken)
- Propranolol (Inderal)
- Timolol (Blocadren)

Drugs that combine both alpha and beta blockage are listed on page 194.

If you have liver or kidney problems, your choice of a beta blocker may be limited. Beta blockers are broken down in your liver or in your kidneys or in both organs. If, for example, your kidneys aren't functioning properly, a beta blocker that's normally removed by your kidneys may build to toxic levels.

Side effects and cautions

Beta blockers have more-frequent side effects than other blood pressure medications, which may be a cause of con-

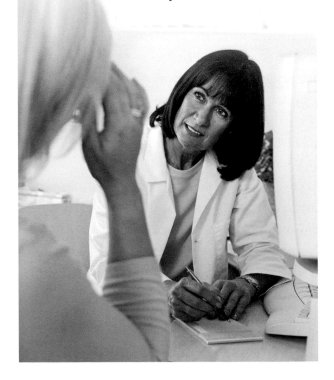

cern. However, many people who take the drugs are bothered only minimally, or the side effects diminish over time.

Two notable side effects are fatigue and the reduced capacity for strenuous physical activity. Other side effects may include cold hands, trouble sleeping, impotence, loss of sex drive, increased risk of diabetes, slight increase in your triglyceride level and slight decrease in your high-density lipoprotein (HDL or "good") cholesterol level.

Beta blockers aren't the first choice of treatment if you're an active person or athlete because they can limit your ability to be fully active. The drugs also aren't recommended if you have asthma or severe blockage in the conducting system of your heart.

ACE inhibitors

Angiotensin-converting enzyme (ACE) inhibitors help reduce blood pressure by preventing the enzyme from producing angiotensin II. This substance causes your blood vessels to contract and stimulates release of the hormone aldosterone (see an illustration of the process on page 24).

Limiting the action of the angiotensin-converting enzyme also allows another substance called bradykinin (brad-e-KI-nin) — which keeps your blood vessels dilated — to remain in your bloodstream, reducing blood pressure.

ACE inhibitors are a common choice among doctors for treating high blood pressure because they're effective and produce few side effects. Among blacks, ACE inhibitors are most effective when combined with a diuretic.

ACE inhibitors offer benefits beyond lowering blood pressure. They help prevent and treat cardiovascular disease, including coronary artery disease, left ventricular hypertrophy, heart failure and stroke. ACE inhibitors also delay progression of kidney disease and may protect against diabetes.

ACE inhibitors include:
- Benazepril (Lotensin)
- Captopril (Capoten)
- Enalapril (Vasotec)
- Fosinopril (Monopril)
- Lisinopril (Prinivil, Zestril)
- Moexipril (Univasc)
- Perindopril (Aceon)
- Quinapril (Accupril)
- Ramipril (Altace)
- Trandolapril (Mavik)

Side effects and cautions

ACE inhibitors generally cause few side effects, but some people who take them develop a dry cough. This occurs more commonly in women than in men. In some people, the cough can be persistent and annoying enough to warrant switching to another medication. ACE inhibitors may also elevate your potassium level, which can be dangerous if the level rises too high.

Other possible side effects may include rash, altered sense of taste and reduced appetite. If you have severe kidney disease, an ACE inhibitor should be used with caution because it can contribute to kidney failure. They aren't recommended if you're pregnant or plan to become pregnant because they can cause birth defects. Rarely — but more commonly in blacks and in smokers — the medication may cause small areas of tissue swelling (angioedema). This can be a potentially life-threatening condition if the swelling occurs in the throat, obstructing breathing.

Angiotensin II receptor blockers

As their name implies, angiotensin II receptor blockers (ARBs) block the action of the chemical angiotensin II — whereas ACE inhibitors block the formation of angiotensin II (see page 24).

I'm afraid of medication side effects. What can I do?

Because certain side effects are associated with a medication doesn't guarantee that you'll experience them. These signs and symptoms are generally reported among only a small number of users. Discuss any concerns you may have with your doctor. There are ways to test your reaction to a drug, for example, by starting at a low dose and gradually raising the dose. Also, many side effects tend to subside after a short amount of use.

Angiotensin II receptor blockers are also different from ACE inhibitors in that they don't affect levels of bradykinin in your bloodstream.

Studies indicate that ARBs are about equally effective as ACE inhibitors in treating high blood pressure and heart failure. They've also been shown to be more effective in treating advanced kidney failure. ARBs can be used to treat cardiovascular disease, including coronary artery disease and stroke. They provide the extra benefit of rarely causing a dry cough.

Angiotensin II receptor blockers include:
- Candesartan (Atacand)
- Eprosartan (Teveten)
- Irbesartan (Avapro)
- Losartan (Cozaar)
- Olmesartan (Benicar)
- Telmisartan (Micardis)
- Valsartan (Diovan)

Side effects and cautions

Side effects are uncommon, but in some people ARBs can cause dizziness, nasal congestion, diarrhea, indigestion and insomnia. In rare cases the medication may cause localized tissue swelling (angioedema).

Like ACE inhibitors, these drugs should be taken with caution if you have severe kidney disease, and not at all if you're pregnant or contemplating pregnancy.

Renin inhibitor

In 2007, the Food and Drug Administration (FDA) announced its approval of aliskiren (Tekturna) as a treatment of hypertension. Aliskiren reduces the ability of the enzyme renin to initiate the process that produces angiotensin II. The drug affects the process at a much earlier stage than do other drugs (see page 24).

Various studies have demonstrated the effectiveness of aliskiren, although results indicate that blacks tend to have smaller reductions in blood pressure than do whites. Results also show that the drug is most effective when used in combination with other medications, especially with a diuretic.

Side effects are uncommon but include diarrhea and an allergic reaction that causes face swelling and difficulty breathing. Don't use aliskiren if you're pregnant or contemplating pregnancy.

Calcium channel blockers

Calcium channel blockers — also called calcium antagonists — work by affecting the muscle cells in the walls of your arteries. These muscle cells contain tiny passages in their membranes called calcium channels. When calcium carried in your bloodstream flows into them, the muscle cells contract and your arteries narrow. Calcium channel blockers prevent the calcium from getting into the muscle cells by blocking the channels.

The drugs don't, however, affect the levels of calcium used by your body to build bone and maintain your musculoskeletal system.

Calcium channel blockers are effective and generally well tolerated. They may work better for blacks than do drugs such as beta blockers, ACE inhibitors and angiotensin II receptor blockers.

Some calcium channel blockers have the added benefit of slowing your heart rate, potentially reducing blood pressure, relieving angina and controlling irregular heartbeat. They can also help prevent migraines and Raynaud's disease, which affects the circulation of blood in your hands and feet.

Types of calcium channel blockers

The two types of calcium channel blockers are determined by the length of time these drugs are effective in your circulatory system:

Short-acting. This type of calcium channel blocker lowers your blood pressure rapidly, often within a mere half-hour. But the effect lasts for only a few hours.

Short-acting calcium channel blockers aren't recommended for treating chronic high blood pressure because it would require you to take the drug three or four times a day. This generally results in poor control of your blood pressure. Some studies have linked the short-acting forms to increased risk of heart attack and sudden cardiac death.

Long-acting. These drugs are absorbed into your body at a much slower rate than the short-acting drugs are. Although it takes them longer to lower your blood pressure, they control the pressure for a longer period of time.

Studies combining data from randomized trials have found long-acting calcium channel blockers aren't as effective as diuretics and beta blockers at controlling blood pressure. Compared with ACE inhibitors, calcium channel blockers are less effective at reducing heart attacks and kidney failure, but more effective at reducing stroke.

The Antihypertensive and Lipid-Lowering Treatment to Prevent Heart Attack Trial (ALLHAT), referred to earlier, confirmed that diuretics were more effective than calcium channel blockers at lowering blood pressure and preventing heart failure.

The various long-acting calcium channel blockers used for treating high blood pressure include:
- Amlodipine (Norvasc)
- Diltiazem (Cardizem, Dilacor XR, others)*
- Felodipine (Plendil)
- Isradipine (DynaCirc CR)
- Nicardipine (Cardene)
- Nifedipine (Adalat, Procardia)
- Nisoldipine (Sular)
- Verapamil (Calan, Covera, others)*

These drugs also slow your heart rate and are useful in treating certain heart arrhythmias and angina, and in preventing second heart attacks and migraines.

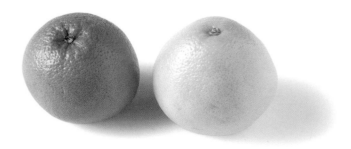

Side effects and cautions

Possible side effects include constipation, headache, rapid heartbeat, rash, swollen feet and lower legs, and swollen gums.

You shouldn't consume grapefruit, grapefruit juice, sour oranges or pomelos if you're taking felodipine, nifedipine, nisoldipine or verapamil. A substance in the juice of these fruits seems to impair the breakdown (metabolism) of the calcium channel blockers, allowing the drugs to build up in your body and become toxic.

Alpha blockers

Alpha blockers lower your blood pressure by reducing the effect of the hormone norepinephrine (noradrenaline), which stimulates muscles in the walls of your smaller arteries. As a result, the walls don't narrow (constrict) as much as they might normally. For older men with prostate problems, alpha blockers also improve urine flow and reduce the number of awakenings at night to go to the bathroom.

Alpha blockers have been used to treat high blood pressure for more than two decades. They're no longer prescribed alone as monotherapy but rather are more appropriate in combination with other high blood pressure drugs.

The National Heart, Lung, and Blood Institute (NHLBI) recommends that people taking alpha blockers should consult their doctors regarding the benefits and disadvantages of using this type of medication.

Alpha blockers, available in both short-acting and long-acting forms, include:
- Doxazosin (Cardura), a long-acting drug
- Prazosin (Minipress), a short-acting drug
- Terazosin (Hytrin), a long-acting drug

Side effects and cautions

These drugs are generally well tolerated. However, when you first begin taking the drug or if you're older, it can cause you to feel dizzy or faint when you stand up. That's because alpha blockers slow the time it takes your body to respond to natural changes in blood pressure when you move from a

Alpha-beta blockers

Certain drugs combine the effects of an alpha blocker and a beta blocker. Alpha-beta blockers such as carvedilol (Coreg) and labetalol (Trandate) are able to lower blood pressure by effectively reducing your heart rate and relaxing your artery walls. The same precautions are necessary for these drugs as for beta blockers and alpha blockers. Possible side effects include fatigue, dizziness, lightheadedness, slow heartbeat, increase in blood sugar and eye dryness.

sitting or lying position to a standing position. Other possible side effects include headache, pounding heartbeat, nausea and weakness.

Central-acting agents

Unlike other blood pressure medications that work primarily on your heart and blood vessels, central-acting agents work on your nervous system. They prevent centers in your brain from signaling your nerves to speed up your heart rate and narrow your blood vessels. As a result, your heart doesn't pump as hard and your blood flows more easily through your arteries.

These medications, also called central adrenergic (ad-ren-UR-jik) inhibitors, aren't used as often as they once were because they can produce strong side effects. However, they're still prescribed in certain circumstances. Your doctor may recommend a central-acting agent to reduce symptoms if you're prone to panic attacks, you have hot flashes or incidents of low blood sugar, or you're going through alcohol or drug withdrawal.

One central-acting agent, clonidine, is available as a skin patch, which is helpful if you have trouble taking pills. Another agent, methyldopa, is often recommended to pregnant women with high blood pressure to lower risks to themselves and the baby.

Central-acting agents include:
- Clonidine (Catapres)
- Guanabenz (Wytensin)
- Guanadrel (Hylorel)*
- Guanfacine (Tenex)
- Methyldopa
- Reserpine*

Drugs that work primarily on the peripheral nervous system outside of the brain.

Side effects and cautions

These drugs can produce extreme fatigue, drowsiness, dizziness or sedation. They can also cause impotence, dry mouth, weight gain, impaired thinking and psychological problems, including depression.

Stopping the use of some central-acting agents can cause your blood pressure to increase rapidly to dangerously high levels. If you're bothered by side effects and want to quit taking the drug, consult your doctor on how to gradually taper its use.

Direct vasodilators

These potent medications are used primarily to treat high blood pressure that doesn't respond well to other medications. They work directly on muscles in your artery walls, preventing the arteries from narrowing.

Direct vasodilators include:
- Hydralazine
- Minoxidil

Side effects and cautions

Common side effects include fast heartbeat, dizziness and fluid retention — none of which is desirable if you have high blood pressure. That's why doctors typically prescribe direct

Working in combination

Two medications may be mixed together into the same tablet or capsule. Examples of these combination drugs are listed below.

Combinations of beta blocker and diuretic:

- Atenolol and chlorthalidone (Tenoretic)
- Bisoprolol and hydrochlorothiazide (Ziac)
- Metoprolol and hydrochlorothiazide (Lopressor HCT)
- Nadolol and bendroflumethiazide (Corzide)
- Propranolol and hydrochlorothiazide (Inderide LA)

Combinations of ACE inhibitor and diuretic:

- Benazepril and hydrochlorothiazide (Lotensin HCT)
- Captopril and hydrochlorothiazide (Capozide)
- Enalapril and hydrochlorothiazide (Vasoretic)
- Lisinopril and hydrochlorothiazide (Prinzide, Zestoretic)

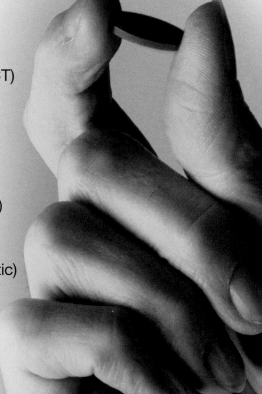

vasodilators with a beta blocker and diuretic, which can reduce the incidence of these symptoms. Other side effects may include gastrointestinal problems, headache, nasal congestion and swelling of your gums. Taking Minoxidil also may result in excessive hair growth. Hydralazine taken in large doses can increase your risk of lupus, an autoimmune disorder that affects your connective tissues.

Combination drug therapy

Approximately half the people with stage 1 high blood pressure can control their blood pressure with just one drug. If this drug isn't effective, your doctor may increase the dosage, provided you aren't experiencing any sig-

Combinations of ARB and diuretic:

- Losartan and hydrochlorothiazide (Hyzaar)
- Valsartan and hydrochlorothiazide (Diovan HCT)

Combinations of two diuretics:

- Amiloride and hydrochlorothiazide (Moduretic)
- Spironolactone and hydrochlorothiazide (Aldactazide)
- Triamterene and hydrochlorothiazide (Dyazide, Maxzide)

Combinations of calcium channel blocker and ACE inhibitor:

- Amlodipine and benazepril (Lotrel)
- Felodipine and enalapril (Lexxel)
- Verapamil and trandolapril (Tarka)

Combination of ARB and calcium channel blocker:

- Valsartan and amlodipine (Exforge)

nificant side effects, or try a completely different drug. Another option your doctor may consider is to add a second drug to the one you're already taking — an approach known as combination drug therapy.

By using a combination of two or more drugs, doctors can typically increase the number of people who respond positively to high blood pressure medication. Your doctor looks for two medications that will enhance each other's effectiveness or reduce side effects, for example, combining a thiazide diuretic — which can lower your potassium level — with a potassium-sparing diuretic, which retains the mineral.

A different example is the combination drug Caduet, which combines amlodipine, a calcium channel blocker, with atorvastatin, a statin used to treat high cholesterol. Since high blood pressure and high cholesterol are often present in the same individual, both disorders can be treated conveniently with a single medication.

Another benefit of combination drugs is that you may be using them at lower doses. For example, certain blood pressure medications, such as thiazide diuretics and beta blockers, increase

the risk of new onset diabetes when used at higher doses or for long duration. The use of these drugs at lower doses in combination with another medication can neutralize this risk, especially if the potassium is kept normal, in controlling high blood pressure.

If, following the onset of therapy using one drug, your blood pressure still exceeds the target goal by more than 20/10 mm Hg — which would include all individuals with stage 2 high blood pressure — the doctor may initiate a new therapy combining two drugs, usually a diuretic and the initial drug. (Generally, if a diuretic isn't the first drug that's prescribed, it's often the second used in combination.)

If you have another medical condition and your blood pressure goal is lower than 130/80 mm Hg, you may need three or more medications. For more on these conditions, see Chapter 5.

Emergency medications

If your blood pressure reaches a dangerously high level, it may be necessary to reduce it rapidly to avoid serious damage to your organs, and even death. Other risks include heart attack, heart failure, stroke, sudden blindness or a rupture in the wall of your aorta.

During blood pressure emergencies, doctors inject a blood pressure lowering medication directly into your bloodstream. The goal is to lower your pressure in progressive, controlled stages. Reducing your blood pressure too fast can have serious, even fatal, consequences.

The initial step is to lower your blood pressure by 25 percent within several minutes to two hours. Once the pressure is reduced by 25 percent, the goal is to lower your blood pressure to near 160/100 millimeters of mercury (mm Hg) within six hours.

Injectable medications used in hypertensive emergencies include:
- Vasodilators, such as fenoldopam, nicardipine hydrochloride, nitro-glycerin, sodium nitroprusside and hydralazine
- Alpha and beta blockers, such as phentolamine, esmolol and labetalol
- The ACE inhibitor enalaprilat

Finding the right medication

Due to the many variables that can affect your blood pressure, finding the right medication or combination of medications is often a trial-and-error process. That's because the doctor must consider everyone's unique physiological makeup, lifestyle and healthy behaviors, and test the impact of different and ever-changing environments.

Nevertheless, almost everyone who takes blood pressure medications is eventually able to come up with a drug regimen that will help achieve his or her target goal. These drugs will allow the individual to feel good and to be fully active. And they will produce few, if any, side effects. In addition to the efficacy of the drug at lowering blood pressure and reducing health risks, your doctor also will consider:

Your tolerance to the drug. If taking a certain medication produces side effects that are unpleasant to live with, such as impotence or headache, then it's probably not the best drug for you. In fact, the medication's side effects may seem worse to live with than your high blood pressure — which generally produces no symptoms.

But don't stop taking a medication without your doctor's guidance. Some drugs need to be tapered off gradually to prevent a rebound of your high blood pressure.

Your compliance with the prescription. If a certain medication is complicated to take and you have a busy schedule, you may forget to take it or simply choose to skip one dose. Because it's vital that you take your medication in the proper manner and at the correct times, the drug your doctor prescribes should be able to fit within your lifestyle. In most cases, it's possible to find a medication or combination medication that you take just once daily.

Your ability to pay for the medication. A drug doesn't do you any good if you can't take it regularly because you can't afford it. Let your doctor know if you can't pay for your medication. Note that very often with drug combinations, there may be fewer copayments on prescription renewals.

? How can I reduce my medication costs?

Following a healthy lifestyle program can reduce the number of medications or the dosage required to reach and maintain your blood pressure goals. Often, after medications have helped control your blood pressure for some months, it may be possible to slowly taper down on the dosage — but do this only under your doctor's guidance. Talk with your doctor about generic equivalent medications. It may also be possible to receive assistance with cost from the manufacturer. For more on cost savings, see Chapter 4.

On the horizon

Beyond the influence they have on your risk of disease, your genes can affect how you respond to medication, including drug therapy for high blood pressure. If promising gene research is successful, it may lead to the development of new drugs.

This research may also assist in the decisions regarding your treatment program. By knowing your genetic makeup, your doctor may be able to make a better selection of drugs to suit your needs and determine the type of medication that's most likely to be effective and beneficial for you.

For example, a team of researchers, including doctors at Mayo Clinic, have identified a gene (GNB3) that may play a role in how people respond to the actions of certain diuretics. They have found that people with one variation of the gene responded better to the medication and had lower blood pressures than did people with another variation of the gene.

Other researchers at Mayo Clinic are currently studying the genetic basis for salt sensitivity. They're looking for the reasons why blood pressure is affected by dietary sodium in some individuals but not in others. Because this salt sensitivity runs in families, the researchers are attempting to find which genes may drive this variability.

New blood pressure drugs are continually being developed, tested and put on the market. Nebivolol is a medication currently under review. It's a new type of beta blocker that is cardioselective — it helps regulate your heart rate and slows it down — but also has qualities that are noncardioselective — it affects your circulatory system by dilating the blood vessels, allowing blood to flow with less force.

Also on the way is a new class of drugs known as endothelin receptor antagonists. These are very strong compounds that relax blood vessels, reducing blood pressure. Ambrisentan (Letairis) is a drug in this class that was approved in 2007 for the treatment of pulmonary arterial hypertension.

Another drug, darusentan, is moving into a Phase 3 clinical trial for the treatment of resistant hypertension, which is high blood pressure that's difficult to control, even following extended treatment with medications.

An implantable device is under study that's designed to help people with severe resistant hypertension. The Rheos Baroreflex Hypertension Therapy System includes pulse generators that are implanted on the carotid arteries — the two major arteries that carry blood from the heart to the brain. The pulse generators stimulate baroreceptors located on the arteries (see page 23), which signal your brain to adjust your blood pressure to within a normal range. This device is not yet approved for commercial sale.

Wrap-up

Key points to remember:
- Medication may be necessary if lifestyle changes aren't effective, you have stage 2 high blood pressure or you have another medical condition that could benefit from drug use.
- While many people can control their blood pressure with just one drug, others need a combination of two or three drugs.
- A diuretic, ACE inhibitor or calcium channel blocker is often prescribed for uncomplicated high blood pressure because of their proven success. Beta blockers are being used less now than before as a single drug for high blood pressure but more for certain conditions that may accompany the disorder.
- Most people taking blood pressure medication are bothered only minimally by side effects.
- Finding the right drug or combination of drugs to control your blood pressure is a process that requires time and patience.

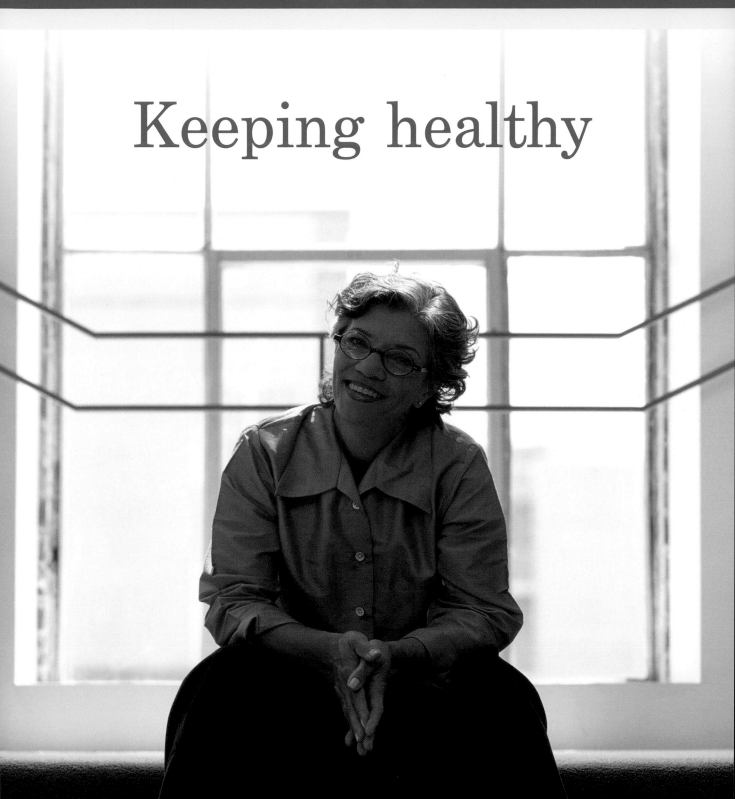

Part 3

Keeping healthy

Chapter 4

Living well with high blood pressure

High blood pressure isn't an illness you can treat and then ignore. It's a condition that you'll need to manage for the rest of your life.

Sometimes this can be difficult because, with high blood pressure, you typically can't feel or see that anything is wrong. With many diseases, such as arthritis or allergies, the symptoms motivate you to treat the condition. You feel the flaring pain and stiffness of arthritic joints or you experience the sneezing and itchy eyes of an allergy attack. You're motivated to take care of the disease because you want those bothersome symptoms to just go away.

The lack of symptoms is why people with high blood pressure often don't take proper steps to treat their disease. It's also why only about one-third of Americans with high blood pressure have the condition under control.

Many others may pretend that they have little to worry about. Despite good advice from their doctors, they can go about their everyday lives and whether or not they stick to their treatment programs seems to make little difference — until organ damage and serious complications have occurred. That's why high blood pressure is often called the "silent killer."

Participating in your health care and managing your high blood pressure — measuring your blood pressure at home, taking your medications properly, maintaining a healthy diet and exercise program, scheduling regular visits to your doctor — are essential. These efforts can significantly increase your chances for living a longer, healthier life, despite high blood pressure.

Taking your blood pressure at home

The doctor's office isn't the only place to measure your blood pressure. Often, you're required to do it by yourself at home. Home monitoring allows you to track your blood pressure in daily circumstances quite apart from a medical office or hospital visit. The record you compile often is a vital asset to the program that's been developed to treat your blood pressure.

If your blood pressure is well controlled, you only may need to check it at home a few days each month. Take two readings in the morning and two in the evening on a day that you're

working, and two pairs of readings on a day that you're relaxing. If you're just starting home monitoring, if you're making changes in medications, or if you have other health problems, you may need to check it more often.

Guidelines from the National Heart, Lung, and Blood Institute (see pages 77-80) advise that you keep your systolic pressure below 140 millimeters of mercury (mm Hg) and diastolic pressure below 90 mm Hg.

But your blood pressure at home is usually slightly lower than it is in a medical setting, typically by a meas-

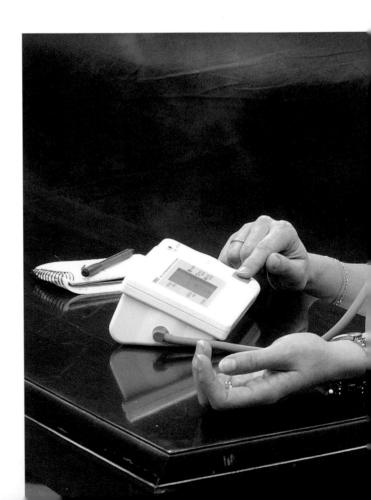

urement of about 5 points. Therefore, your readings at home should have an average systolic pressure below 135 mm Hg and an average diastolic pressure below 85 mm Hg. If a lower goal is set for your office blood pressure, discuss with your doctor what the goal at home should be.

Benefits of home monitoring

Measuring your blood pressure at home can help:

Track the progress of your treatment. Because high blood pressure has no

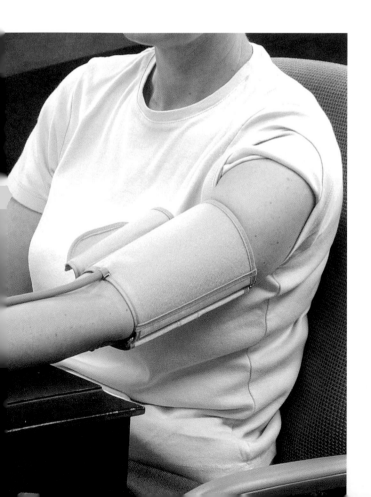

symptoms, the only way to make sure lifestyle changes or medications are working is to check your blood pressure regularly. Monitoring your blood pressure at home provides vital information between medical visits that you can share with your doctor.

Promote better control. Taking responsibility for measuring your blood pressure tends to motivate you in other areas of your program. It can give you added incentive to eat a better diet, increase your activity level and take your medication properly.

Identify your usual blood pressure. For some people, simply going to a doctor's office causes their blood pressure to temporarily increase to a high level. For others, the opposite happens — their blood pressure drops during doctor appointments (see page 68). Home monitoring can help identify or confirm your usual blood pressure.

Save money. Home monitoring saves you the cost of going to your doctor's office every time you need a blood pressure reading. This is especially true when you first start taking medications or your doctor adjusts the dosage. With these changes, frequent measurements help to ensure better control.

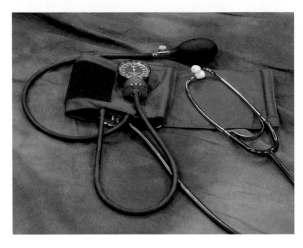

Aneroid monitor

Aneroid blood pressure monitors include a cuff, rubber bulb to inflate the cuff, stethoscope to listen for your pulse, and gauge on which to read your pressure.

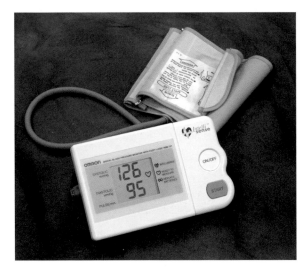

Electronic monitor

Electronic blood pressure monitors include a digital gauge and cuff that inflates at the push of a button.

Types of blood pressure monitors

Not all blood pressure monitors are the same: Some are easier to use, some are more reliable, and some are simply inaccurate and a waste of money. To get an accurate reading, an appropriately sized cuff should be wrapped around your upper arm. It's important that the cuff fits properly. A cuff that's too narrow or too wide won't provide accurate readings.

The inflatable bladder in the cuff should encircle 80 percent to 100 percent of your upper arm and reach three-fourths of the way from your elbow to your shoulder. Ideally, the cuff will have a D-ring fastener to securely close it. Have your doctor measure your arm to determine the appropriate size of the cuff, particularly if you have a large upper arm.

Blood pressure monitors are available in the following forms:

Mercury-column models. These monitors, which look like oversized thermometers, are very accurate and were once the standard monitoring devices. Due to safety and environmental concerns about mercury poisoning and disposal, these devices are being phased out for home use.

Aneroid models. These monitors use metal instead of liquid to measure blood pressure. Attached to the cuff is a round dial that's marked in increments corresponding to 2 millimeters of mercury. During use, the needle on the face of the dial moves to indicate your blood pressure level.

Doctors often recommend aneroid models for use at home because they're inexpensive and easy to transport. In addition, some dials are extra-large for easier reading and some models have a built-in stethoscope, which makes them easier to use.

A disadvantage is that once a year you need to verify the monitor's accuracy by comparing it to a standard device at your doctor's office. If the reading is off by more than 3 millimeters, you should replace the unit.

Standard aneroid monitors aren't recommended if you have trouble hearing or have poor dexterity in your hands. These monitors require listening to the sounds of turbulent blood passing through an artery. They also require using a stethoscope and bulb pump.

Electronic models. Also referred to as digital monitors, these models are the most popular and easiest to use for home monitoring. They also tend to be more expensive than aneroid devices, though their cost continues to decline.

Electronic blood pressure monitors generally require you to do two things — wrap the inflatable cuff around your arm and push a button with your finger. The cuff automatically inflates with air and then slowly deflates. Your blood pressure and heart rate are displayed on the digital gauge.

Unlike aneroid models, electronic monitors detect motion in the artery wall rather than the sound of blood flow. For some people, aneroid and electronic monitors may not give exactly the same measurements.

Electronic monitors are easier to damage than are aneroid devices. As with aneroid models, you need to check the electronic monitor's accuracy at least once a year. If you have an irregular heart rhythm, check with your doctor before buying an electronic model — it may not give you an accurate reading.

Finger or wrist models. To make blood pressure monitors more compact and

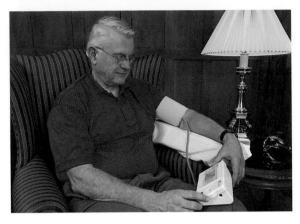

How to do it

Using an electronic model involves sitting with your arm at heart level, placing the cuff around your upper arm, relaxing and pressing a button to inflate the cuff and get a reading.

easy to use, some manufacturers have produced models that measure blood pressure in your wrist or finger, instead of your upper arm. To get an accurate reading at either of these locations, it's very important that your hand and wrist be at heart level. Unfortunately, the technology of finger monitors is not equal to their simplicity of use. Avoid them because they're inaccurate. Wrist monitors also are difficult to calibrate.

Home monitoring tips

Learning to take a blood pressure reading correctly takes a little training and practice, but the monitors are not diffi-

cult to use. A variety of monitors are available at medical supply stores and many pharmacies. After you purchase a monitor, take it with you to your next doctor's visit.

In addition to making sure the device works properly, the doctor or nurse can teach you how to use it and answer your questions. Keep in mind that if you have an irregular heart rhythm, getting an accurate reading from these devices will be more difficult.

To get an accurate reading of your blood pressure:

- Remember that your blood pressure varies throughout the day, and readings are often a little higher in the morning than they are in the afternoon and evening. So don't measure your blood pressure right after you get up in the morning. Wait until after you've been active for an hour or more.
- Take a reading before you eat or wait at least a half-hour after you've eaten, smoked, or used caffeine or alcohol. Food, tobacco, caffeine and alcohol can temporarily increase your blood pressure.
- Go to the bathroom before the reading. A full bladder will slightly increase your blood pressure.

- Sit quietly for three to five minutes before taking a reading.
- Your mood can affect your blood pressure. If you've had a difficult day, don't be alarmed if your blood pressure reflects it.
- Check your blood pressure before you exercise, not afterwards. Your pressure varies the most during and immediately after exercise.

To get an accurate reading, it's important to use proper technique. Follow the 10 steps listed here. If you have an electronic device, some of these steps won't apply. Ask your doctor for additional instructions.

Step 1: Sit comfortably. Keep your legs and ankles uncrossed and your back supported against the back of a chair. Rest your arm at heart level on a table or the arm of a chair. If you're right-handed, you may find it easier to measure pressure in your left arm and vice versa. Be consistent with which arm you use. Take your blood pressure at consistent times, such as always in the morning or in the evening.

Step 2: Locate your pulse in the arm on which you'll place the cuff so that you know where to place the stethoscope. Do this by pressing firmly on the inside of your elbow, above the bend. If you can't find a pulse, you may be pressing either too hard or too soft.

Step 3: Wrap the cuff around your bare arm, not over clothing. Rolling up a

Video demonstration of home monitoring

Visit the High Blood Pressure Center on MayoClinic.com to see a video on how to use home blood pressure monitors. The video shows the proper technique for both aneroid and electronic monitors. To view the video, go to *www.MayoClinic.com,* click High Blood Pressure Center and look for the link "How to monitor your own blood pressure."

sleeve until it tightens around your arm can give you an inaccurate reading, so you may slip your arm out of the sleeve. Place the cuff about 2 inches (5 centimeters) above your elbow bend. The inflatable portion of the cuff should fit snugly around your arm.

Step 4: Place the earpieces of the stethoscope into your ears, with the earpieces facing forward. Place the flat side of the stethoscope directly over your pulse, just under the lower edge of the cuff. If your monitor has a built-in stethoscope, an arrow on the cuff may mark which section should be located over your pulse. If the arterial sounds aren't clearly heard, place the bell side of the stethoscope below the lower edge of the cuff.

Step 5: Put the gauge or digital screen where you can easily read it. Make sure it registers at zero before you inflate the cuff.

Step 6: Using the hand of your uncuffed arm, squeeze the hand bulb repeatedly to pump air into the cuff. Inflate the cuff to about 30 millimeters (mm) above your normal systolic pressure, then stop squeezing. You shouldn't be able to hear your pulse when listening through the stethoscope.

Step 7: Turn the release valve and slowly deflate the cuff at 2 to 3 mm per second. Watch the gauge and listen carefully. When you hear the first tapping sound of your pulse, note the reading on the gauge. If the gauge's needle jerks slightly, use the lowest reading. This is your systolic pressure.

Step 8: Continue deflating the cuff. When the pulse sounds stop, note the gauge's reading. This is your diastolic pressure. For some people, the pulse doesn't disappear, but will fade noticeably. That sudden drop in sound indicates diastolic pressure. Then release the valve completely to deflate the cuff.

Step 9: Wait a minute after the first reading and repeat the procedure to check for accuracy. If you have trouble getting consistent readings, check with your doctor. The problem may be your technique or your equipment. Also contact your doctor if you notice an unusual or persistent increase in your blood pressure.

Step 10: Keep a log of your blood pressure readings. Along with each reading, include the date and time. Bring the log to your next medical appointment to show your doctor. A sample log is shown on page 213.

Date	Time	Systolic pressure	Diastolic pressure	Pulse	Medication changes/comments

Seeing your doctor regularly

It's vital that you schedule regular checkups with your doctor to make sure you're getting your blood pressure under control and your treatment program is progressing with no serious side effects or complications.

Unfortunately, close to half the people with high blood pressure don't visit their doctor on a regular basis. This may be yet another reminder of why so many Americans with high blood pressure have so much difficulty controlling their condition.

If you have stage 1 high blood pressure and no evidence of organ damage, the doctor likely will want to see you again within one to two months after you start a treatment program.

During that first follow-up visit, your doctor will evaluate your progress, determine if your blood pressure has decreased, ask how efforts are going to change your lifestyle and check if there are any side effects to the medications you're taking. If your blood pressure hasn't decreased, your doctor may adjust your program.

If you have stage 2 high blood pressure and other medical problems that com-

? Will I be able to stop taking blood pressure medication?

You've taken your medication faithfully, and your blood pressure is within a normal range again. Now you're wondering if one day you'll be able to stop using drugs. The most likely answer is no.

Some people with high blood pressure that's well controlled are able to reduce the amount of medication they take daily. However, most people continue to take some medication for the rest of their lives. Blood pressure drugs ensure that your blood pressure stays at safe levels and can lower your risk of complications from uncontrolled hypertension — including stroke, heart attack, heart failure, kidney failure and dementia.

In a few cases, people with stage 1 high blood pressure who have maintained a normal blood pressure for at least a year can discontinue their medication. But to do this, your doctor needs to set up a plan for gradually reducing the medication. He or she will also want to see you frequently to make sure your blood pressure doesn't increase again as you wean yourself from the drug.

To successfully manage your blood pressure without medication, controlling your weight, staying active, eating well, avoiding tobacco and limiting alcohol are essential. Some people who successfully taper off blood pressure drugs eventually need to go back on medication.

If unpleasant side effects are the main reason why you want to discontinue your medication, a better solution may be to work with your doctor to reduce or eliminate these side effects.

plicate your treatment, you may need to see your doctor more frequently — perhaps every two to four weeks until your blood pressure is under control.

Once your blood pressure is well controlled, a visit to your doctor once or twice a year is often all that's needed, unless you have a coexisting medical condition, such as diabetes, high cholesterol, or heart or kidney disease. Then, you'll need to see your doctor more frequently.

Follow-up visits typically involve measuring your blood pressure twice, undergoing a general physical examination and having some routine tests. The tests can alert your doctor to possible problems resulting from medication or to a decline in your heart or kidney function related to high blood pressure. Follow-up visits are also a good time to talk with your doctor about issues related to your weight, diet, and activity level, as well as other efforts to improve your lifestyle.

If your blood pressure doesn't match the target goal you've set, you may be tempted to give up the program. But don't. Instead, discuss with your doctor why the plan may not be working and consider the adjustments you can make. Reaching a target goal may simply take more time. You can help by:

- Learning all you can about high blood pressure
- Practicing good lifestyle habits, such as controlling your weight, eating well, being physically active, not smoking, limiting alcohol and managing stress
- Reviewing medications and supplements you're taking, both prescription and over-the-counter
- Being optimistic and patient
- Seeking out a high blood pressure specialist if you feel your treatment plan isn't helping

Avoiding drug interactions

The effectiveness of your medication depends in large part on you. When, how and with what you take your pills are important factors.

Taking medications correctly

You need to take your medications exactly as prescribed to get the best results. That may sound obvious, but

Nutritional and herbal supplements

Alternative health practices and products are becoming increasingly popular, but they aren't always effective or safe. If you're taking a supplement — or considering using one — talk with your doctor about it.

Supplements promoted to lower blood pressure

Coenzyme Q10	Study results are inconclusive on whether it controls blood pressure.
Cola nut	Has effect of increasing blood pressure.
Fish oil capsules containing omega-3 fatty acids	Capsules are high in fat and calories. May produce gastrointestinal side effects, leave fishy aftertaste. Better to eat fish, although some fish contain high levels of mercury.
Garlic	Study results are mixed. No conclusive evidence it controls blood pressure.
Ginkgo	No conclusive evidence it controls blood pressure.
Green tea	No conclusive evidence it controls blood pressure.
Potassium, calcium and magnesium	May interfere with other medications. Magnesium supplements may cause diarrhea. Excessive potassium can interfere with heart rhythm.
Vitamin C	No conclusive evidence it controls blood pressure.

Supplements that can increase blood pressure

Ephedra (ephedrine)	Claims to promote weight loss, provide herbal high. Avoid. Banned by Food and Drug Administration. Similar compounds include bitter orange (Citrus aurantium).
Licorice	Claims to cure ulcers, coughs and colds. Avoid. Can increase blood pressure.
Yohimbe	Claims to increase sexual desire. Avoid. Can increase blood pressure.

by some estimates only half the people taking blood pressure medications do so in correct doses at correct times.

If you take your pills too early, you increase the level of the drug in your bloodstream. This overdose can produce symptoms and side effects such as nausea and diarrhea.

If you take your pills too late or forget to take them, your blood pressure may increase as the drug levels decrease. And if you stop taking your pills entirely, your blood pressure may rebound to levels that are higher than before your condition was diagnosed.

It's important to know the names and doses of all of the medications you take. To help you remember, keep a list in your purse or wallet and update it when necessary. Keep the original containers. Periodically take them to your doctor to make sure you're taking the right drug in the proper dosage.

Here are other tips to help you take your medication properly:

Use daily activities as reminders. If you take a morning medication, put the pills near your breakfast dishes, toothbrush or razor — so long as it doesn't endanger children or pets — or put a sticker near these items to remind you to take your pills.

Set a clock or wristwatch alarm. The alarm will remind you when it's time to take your medication.

Use a pillbox. If you take several drugs, purchase a pillbox with compartments for each day of the week. Load the box once a week to keep track of which pills you take and when.

Ask for help from a loved one. Ask a family member or trusted friend to remind you to take your pills, at least until you've integrated the habit into your daily routine.

Take pills with water. Water helps dissolve the drug. If you generally take your pills with another liquid, check with the doctor or pharmacist to make sure it mixes well with the medication.

If you're supposed to take your pills with food, do so. Otherwise the drug may not be absorbed properly into your bloodstream.

Use good lighting. Don't take your medication in the dark. You might unintentionally take the wrong pill.

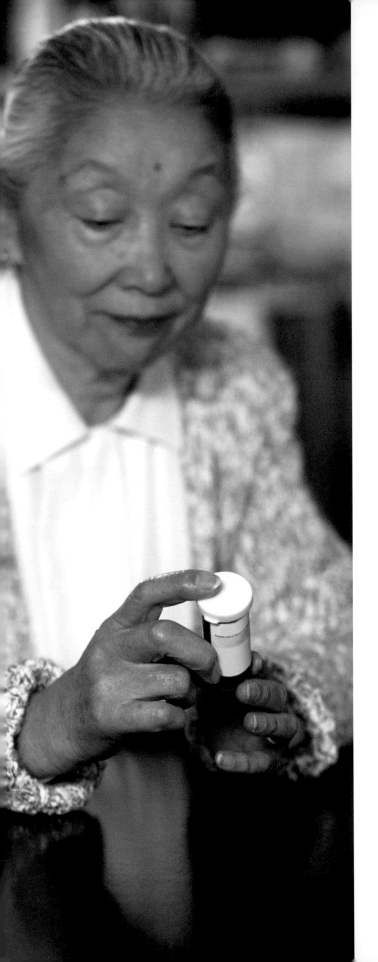

Note any side effects. Provide this information to your doctor at your next checkup. Your doctor may adjust the dosage or try a different medication. Many blood pressure drugs can produce side effects. However, with the right medication, most people experience few problems.

Refill your prescriptions in advance. Plan to resupply at least a couple of weeks ahead, in case the unexpected upsets your routine. Snowstorms, the flu and accidents are just a few examples of surprises that can delay your trip to the pharmacy.

Don't change your dosage. If your blood pressure increases even though you're taking your medication properly, don't increase the dosage on your own. Talk with your doctor first. Similarly, don't decrease your dosage without first consulting your doctor.

Preventing interactions

There are many medications that can be used to control high blood pressure. Some produce dangerous side effects if they're mixed with other prescription drugs, over-the-counter (OTC) medicines, nutritional and herbal supplements, illicit drugs, and even some foods. So it's important that you tell your doctor about all of the medications you're taking and to ask about any potentially harmful interactions.

Prescription drugs. Many prescription drugs can interfere with certain blood pressure medications. Some prescription drugs, such as sibutramine (Meridia), can actually increase blood pressure in some people.

Many common anti-inflammatory drugs can interfere with at least four different classes of blood pressure medications: diuretics, beta blockers, angiotensin-converting enzyme (ACE) inhibitors and angiotensin II receptor blockers (ARBs).

They counteract the effects of diuretics by causing your body to retain sodium and fluid. They counteract the effects of beta blockers by preventing the production of chemicals that relax blood vessels. And they reduce the ability of ACE inhibitors and ARBs to widen blood vessels. Their effect on a new class of drug, direct renin inhibitors, hasn't yet been studied.

If you're taking a prescription medication, your doctor can adjust the dose of your blood pressure medication to counteract any negative effects. Problems most often develop with the intermittent use of anti-inflammatory medications, and it's important to tell your doctor if you take such drugs, even occasionally. Your doctor may switch your blood pressure medication to something that's less affected by the prescription drug.

Over-the-counter products. Pain relievers, decongestants and diet pills can pose problems if you're taking blood pressure medication. Some of these OTC products when taken with certain blood pressure drugs may increase your blood pressure.

OTC medications include nonsteroidal anti-inflammatory drugs (NSAIDs) such as adult aspirin (325 milligrams, or mg), ibuprofen (Advil, Motrin, others) and naproxen sodium (Aleve).

Acetaminophen (Tylenol, others) isn't an anti-inflammatory drug, and it doesn't interfere with blood pressure medications. Children's aspirin (81 mg) doesn't affect blood pressure control.

Use cold and allergy products carefully. Read labels to see if they contain a decongestant such as pseudoephedrine or phenylephrine (used in nasal

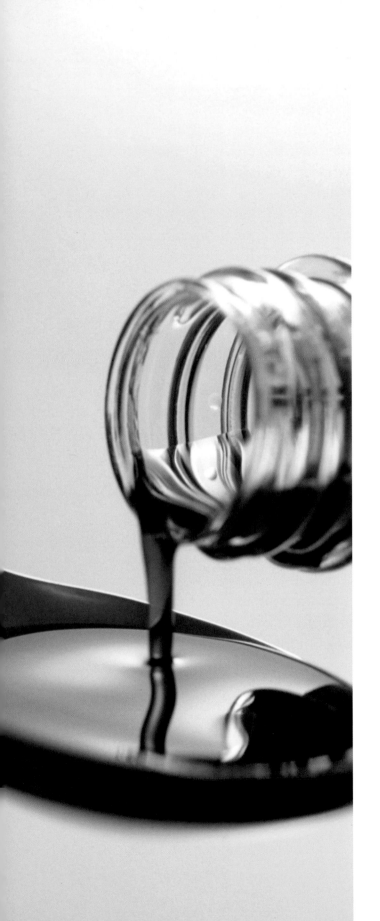

sprays). These compounds relieve congestion by narrowing blood vessels, minimizing blood flow to a localized area. This narrowing of blood vessels can increase your blood pressure. Ask your doctor for guidance.

Illicit drugs. Cocaine narrows and inflames your blood vessels and interferes with the effects of blood pressure medications. Street drugs can also cause dangerous drug interactions.

Food. Grapefruit, grapefruit juice, Seville (sour) oranges and pomelos (a form of grapefruit native to India) can interfere with the ability of your intestinal wall to process certain calcium channel blockers. This causes the drug to build up in your body, which can lead to harmful side effects.

If you take the drugs felodipine (Plendil), nifedipine (Adalat, Procardia) or verapamil (Calan SR, Covera-HS, others), don't eat any of the citrus fruit mentioned above and don't drink grapefruit juice. Sweet oranges and tangerines generally don't interfere with drug absorption.

Natural licorice, the bittersweet ingredient often added to chewing tobacco and some cough drops, can increase your blood pressure because it contains glycyrrhizic acid. This type of acid makes your kidneys retain sodium and fluid. If you take a diuretic to remove excess sodium and fluids, avoid natural licorice. Artificially flavored licorice — the kind often used in candy — isn't a problem.

Reducing medication costs

Many blood pressure medications can become expensive if you have to take a drug every day for the rest of your life — a situation that's magnified if you take two or more drugs daily. However, there are ways you can reduce your medication costs.

Generic drugs. Once a pharmaceutical company's patent on a drug expires — usually after 17 years — other companies are free to make the drug from the same ingredients. This competition often spurs the original supplier to reduce the price. In addition, the cost of the new generic brands is usually lower because generic manufacturers don't have to recoup the costs of research and development.

Ask your doctor if it's OK for you to take a generic drug. And don't be sur-

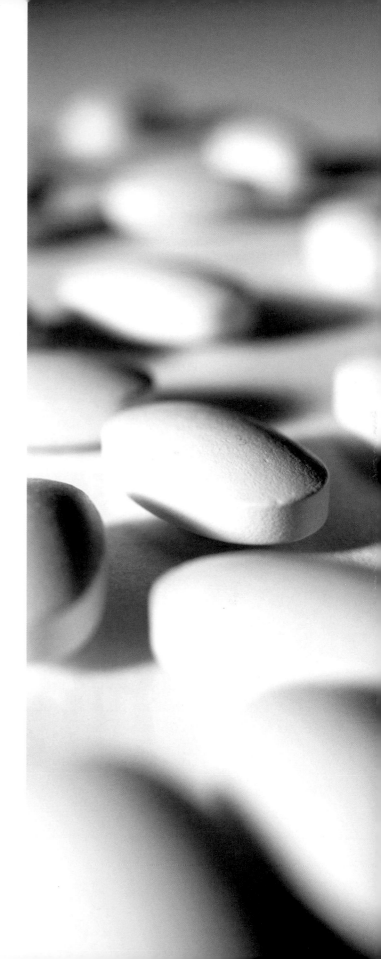

prised if the new pills look different from the original. Generic drugs are often another shape and color. Because of this, read the label carefully to make sure that the dosage is the same as it was for the original drug.

A generic drug doesn't face the same rigorous testing as a new brand-name drug. But the Food and Drug Administration does check to ensure that a generic drug delivers the same amount of active ingredient in the same amount of time as the original brand-name drug.

Generic drugs must also meet the same standards of identity, quality and purity as required for brand-name products. Still, it's a good idea to monitor your blood pressure more frequently when you first start taking a generic drug.

Splitting pills. Pills generally come in several doses. Many times higher dose pills cost only a small amount more than lower dose versions. For example, if your prescription is for 50-milligram (mg) tablets, you can buy 100-mg tablets and split them to save money.

You can purchase an inexpensive pill splitter at medical supply stores and some pharmacies. It's more convenient and accurate than using a knife and a cutting board.

However, not all pills can be split. For example, this technique doesn't work with capsules containing sustained-release granules. The various ingredients aren't evenly distributed within the capsule. Nor should you split pills that are coated to keep them from dissolving in your stomach. Cutting negates the coating's effect.

In addition, the medication you take may not come in a larger dose that can be evenly divided. The pills *must* be cut into equal proportions. If you're taking several medications or you have a condition that makes cutting difficult, pill splitting may become more of a hassle than help.

Check with your doctor or pharmacist before splitting your pills. Make sure it's safe to do so. Even if you do split pills, follow up with your doctor to make sure your medication is working.

Buying in bulk. In addition to comparison shopping for the best buy among pharmacies, also check discount mail-order pharmacies. Their prices may be 10 percent to 35 percent lower than you'll find at some pharmacies. The discount is available because the clearinghouse buys and sells in bulk.

A disadvantage of buying in bulk is that if you stockpile too much of the medication, some of it may reach its expiration date before you can use it. If your doctor changes your prescription, you may also end up with medication you can't use. It's best to buy enough for only three to six months.

Another disadvantage to buying from mail-order suppliers is that you miss having a pharmacist who's familiar with your medical history and all of the medications you're taking. But if you're diligent about keeping your doctors updated on your medications, discount suppliers can provide a safe and wallet-friendly alternative.

Combination drugs. Some blood pressure medications are used together so often that manufacturers have combined the ingredients into single tablets. These combination tablets are usually less expensive than buying the pills individually, and you also save on copayments. If you take more than one blood pressure medication, ask your doctor if the medications come in combination form (see pages 196-197).

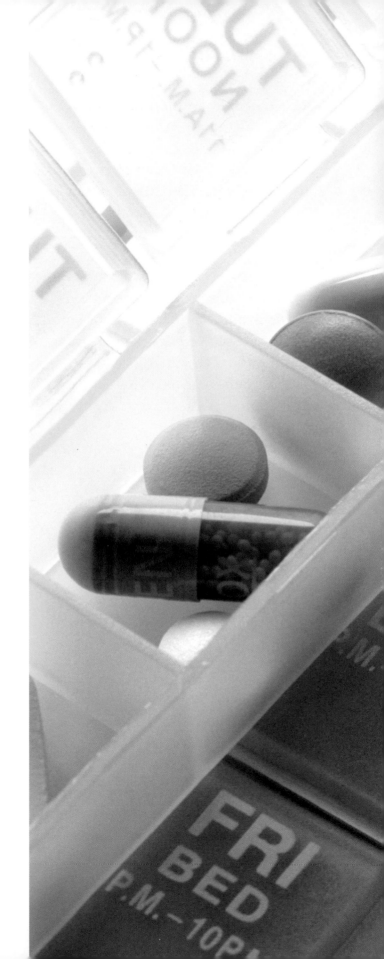

Assistance programs. Some social service organizations and pharmaceutical companies offer free medication or drugs at greatly reduced prices to people facing financial hardship. Your doctor can refer you to the appropriate social services or drug manufacturer.

A directory of assistance programs is available from the Pharmaceutical Research and Manufacturers of America (PhRMA), 950 F St. N.W., Washington, D.C., 20004, (202-835-3400).

Recognizing an emergency

Uncontrolled high blood pressure can gradually erode your health by wearing down many of your body systems and by damaging your organs.

Sometimes, though, blood pressure can rise high enough to suddenly become life-threatening, requiring immediate care. When this happens, it's a hypertensive emergency.

Hypertensive emergencies are rare. They occur when your blood pressure increases to a dangerously high level and is often accompanied by other serious symptoms.

Generally, a reading of 180/110 mm Hg or greater is considered a dangerously high level. If you have another medical condition, lower elevations in your blood pressure also can trigger a hypertensive emergency. The danger level in children is lower, depending on age and height.

Causes of hypertensive emergencies may include:
*   Forgetting to take your blood pressure medication
*   Acute stroke
*   Acute heart attack
*   Heart failure
*   Kidney failure
*   Rupture of the aorta
*   Interaction between medications
*   Postoperative complications
*   Convulsions during pregnancy (eclampsia)

To prevent damage to your organs, your blood pressure needs to be lowered immediately but in controlled stages. Lowering it too fast can interfere with normal blood flow, possibly resulting in too little blood to your heart, brain and other organs.

Emergency warning signs

In addition to dangerously high blood pressure readings, signs and symptoms that often signal a hypertensive emergency include:

- Severe headache, accompanied by confusion and blurred vision
- Severe chest pain
- Marked shortness of breath
- Nausea and vomiting
- Seizures
- Unresponsiveness

Don't drink or eat anything and, if you can, lie down until emergency help arrives or you get to a hospital.

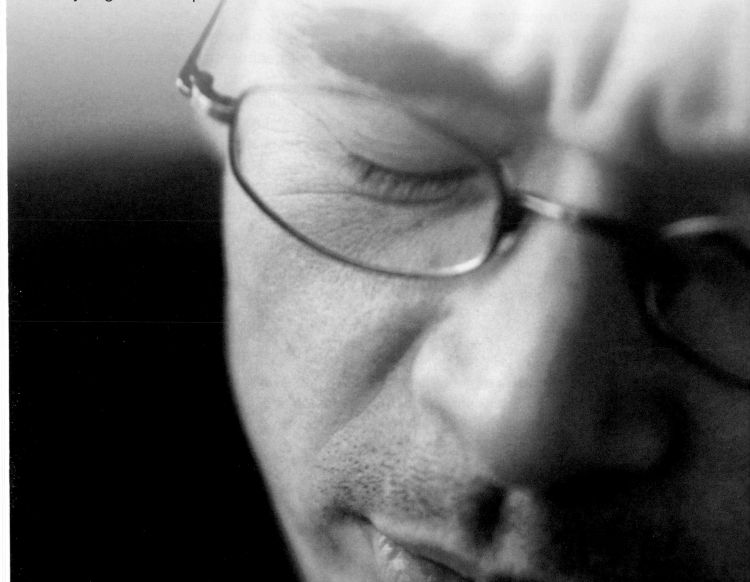

pressure. They're 25 percent more likely to have high blood pressure than are women who don't take HRT.

It's best to discuss the risks and benefits of HRT with your doctor. However, women who take HRT respond to lifestyle changes and medications just as those who don't take HRT.

Prehypertension can be managed with lifestyle programs that aim for a blood pressure of less than 120/80 mm Hg. For women who have heart disease, kidney disease, stroke or diabetes, using medications to lower blood pressure to less than 130/80 mm Hg is often recommended.

Children

Infants are born with low blood pressure that increases quickly during the first month of their life. During childhood, their blood pressure continues to slowly increase into the teenage years, until it has reached a level comparable to that of an adult.

Blood pressure isn't measured routinely in infants and toddlers because it's difficult to get an accurate reading.

However, young children can develop high blood pressure, and just as with adults, it may not always be accompanied by symptoms. The condition may not be suspected until more obvious problems occur, such as unexplained irritability, vomiting, failure to grow properly or, in extreme cases, seizures or heart failure.

When your child reaches age 3, it's appropriate to have his or her blood pressure checked at every well-child visit. To determine whether your child's blood pressure is truly elevated, his or her blood pressure is rated on a percentile basis, taking into account age and height — charts are available that show this information.

At any age, tall children tend to have higher blood pressures than do children who are short or of average height. A child with a blood pressure reading above the 95th percentile is considered to have high blood pressure. A reading between the 90th and 94th percentile would indicate a child with prehypertension.

More often than in adults, high blood pressure in children is associated with a clearly defined cause. Those causes may include narrowing of a kidney artery, kidney failure and hormonal abnormalities. Head trauma, brain infections and tumors also can cause hypertension. Coarctation of the aorta is a narrowing of the main artery from your heart (see page 50). This congenital problem, which causes high blood pressure in the upper part of the body, may escape detection until later in life.

Your doctor will likely perform several tests to try to find a cause for your child's high blood pressure. If all test results are normal and all other possible causes are eliminated, then the child is considered to have essential hypertension. The condition may be related to lifestyle factors such as obesity, poor diet and lack of exercise. If more than one child in a family has high blood pressure, a genetic link may be suspected.

As an increasing number of young children become less physically active and more obese, more of them run the risk of developing high blood pressure in their teens. Between 1 percent and 3 percent of children in the United States have chronic high blood pressure. This percentage appears to increase substantially among children who are overweight or obese — several studies report that being obese nearly triples a

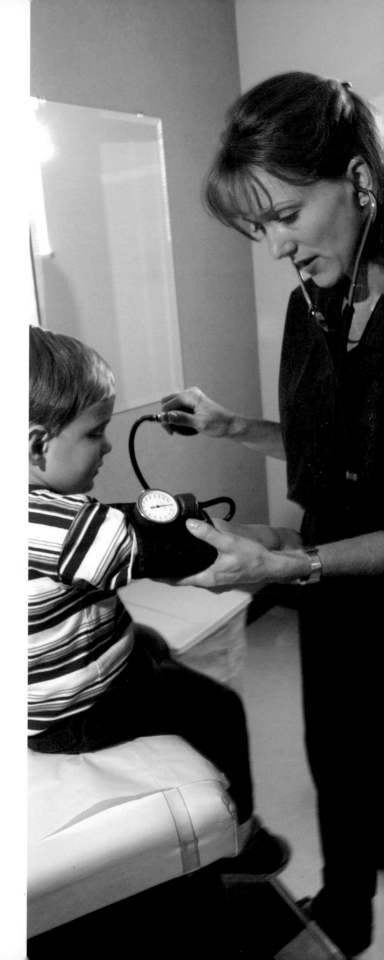

child's chance of having high blood pressure. High cholesterol or other blood fat abnormalities often coexist with high blood pressure and will need management, as well.

For children with essential hypertension, lifestyle changes are commonly recommended. It can be hard for young people to stick to a healthy diet and regular exercise plan, especially for teenagers wanting to control their own lifestyle choices. Casting these goals as family priorities can reinforce the importance of these changes to your child's and your family's future health.

High blood pressure in children that's ignored or uncontrolled can lead to the same kinds of problems as experienced by adults with the condition, including damage to organs such as the heart, brain, eyes and kidneys.

Your doctor may prescribe medication if your child's blood pressure is quite high or if lifestyle changes aren't working. The same medications used to control blood pressure in adults are used for children, only in smaller doses. For information on blood pressure medications, see Step 5 in this book. Some clearly identifiable causes of the condition may be remedied with surgery.

Ethnic groups

Studies examining the prevalence of high blood pressure in America show that the condition affects a disproportionate number of blacks, compared with whites, Hispanics and Asians. Hypertension in blacks also appears to be more likely to develop at a younger age and result in more severe complications than for individuals in most other American ethnic groups.

The reasons for this disparity are unclear, although speculation abounds. But until scientists can determine the basic causes of high blood pressure, explaining differences across populations is likely impossible.

Nonetheless, the risk factors for hypertension — such as obesity, physical inactivity, too much dietary sodium and not enough potassium, excessive alcohol intake, and not eating enough fruits and vegetables — remain the same across all ethnic groups.

With proper medical care, strokes, heart attacks and progressive kidney failure from high blood pressure can be reduced equally as well in blacks as in whites. In addition, black participants in the DASH-Sodium dietary study (see page 88) had the greatest reduction in their blood pressure. Blacks also seem to benefit more than whites from increasing their potassium intake.

At one point, diuretics were considered the most beneficial drug for blacks with hypertension. But recent guidelines recommend combination therapy — such as a diuretic combined with an ACE inhibitor or ARB — for most blacks with hypertension. Combination therapy allows for greater effectiveness in lowering blood pressure and lower doses of each medication, with less risk of side effects.

The prevalence of high blood pressure among some populations of American Indians is higher than in whites. And among Hispanics, Asian-Americans and Pacific Islanders, the incidence of high blood pressure is slightly lower than in whites.

Other conditions

Often, high blood pressure is accompanied by other medical conditions that make it more difficult to treat and control. So if you have another chronic illness in addition to high blood pressure, it's especially important that you see your doctor regularly.

Cardiovascular problems

Cardiovascular conditions that often coexist with hypertension include:

Arrhythmia. High blood pressure can cause your heart to beat in an irregular rhythm. You're at greater risk of developing this condition if your blood contains low levels of potassium or magnesium. This sometimes happens due to treatment if you're taking a diuretic. A high pulse pressure will increase the risk, as well (see page 238).

Controlling your high blood pressure decreases the pressure on your heart's pumping ability and reduces the risk of cardiovascular complications such as the enlargement of your heart's left ventricle. This in turn reduces the likelihood of developing arrhythmia.

To help control or prevent arrhythmia, with your doctor's consent, eat plenty of foods containing potassium and magnesium, such as fresh fruits and vegetables. If this doesn't help, your doctor may recommend that you take supplements to keep your potassium and magnesium levels normal.

Pulse pressure

Pulse pressure is the difference between your systolic pressure and diastolic pressure readings. For example, if your systolic pressure is 120 mm Hg and your diastolic is 80 mm Hg, your pulse pressure is 40. High pulse pressure — more than 50 mm Hg — may be a sign of isolated systolic hypertension (ISH), in which systolic pressure is quite high but diastolic pressure remains normal. A high pulse pressure in older adults increases the risk of cardiovascular disease and stroke. Pulse pressure and the accompanying risks are often reduced with a reduction in systolic pressure.

In addition, taking a fish oil supplement also may help. Fish oil, which is high in omega-3 fatty acids, has been shown to lower risk of sudden death due to arrhythmia. The American Heart Association recommends eating two servings a week of fatty fish to help lower the risk of you developing cardiovascular disease.

Arteriosclerosis and atherosclerosis. Over time, high pressure in your arteries can make the vessel walls thick and stiff — often this development will restrict blood flow. This process is called arteriosclerosis, or hardening of the arteries. Atherosclerosis is a specific type of arteriosclerosis caused by the buildup of fatty plaques in the walls of the arteries (for more information on these conditions, see pages 33-34).

Risk factors in addition to high blood pressure include smoking, abnormal lipids, too much weight, lack of exercise, diabetes and excessive alcohol consumption. Your doctor may ask you to better manage these factors.

Your doctor may also prescribe a low-dose diuretic or beta blocker to reduce the volume of blood. ACE inhibitors and ARBs may help reverse the stiffness in your blood vessels.

Coronary artery disease. High blood pressure often coexists with coronary artery disease. Having high blood pressure puts added force against the walls of your arteries, which can damage the blood vessels and increase your risk of atherosclerosis. Atherosclerosis obstructs blood vessels, including the coronary arteries — your heart's own circulatory system. The inadequate blood flow damages the heart muscle, increasing your risk of chest pain (angina), heart attack and heart failure.

Diuretics, beta blockers, ACE inhibitors, ARBs and aldosterone antagonists are often used to treat people with high blood pressure and coronary artery disease because, in addition to lowering blood pressure, they reduce the risk of heart attack and heart failure. A beta blocker and calcium antagonist may be prescribed to relieve angina and, in some cases, reduce the risk of a second heart attack. Beta blockers have been shown to reduce the amount of atherosclerotic plaques in coronary arteries.

A low-dose regimen of aspirin (81 mg) for people with controlled high blood pressure can help reduce the risk of cardiovascular problems and the recurrence of heart attack and stroke. In cer-

tain cases, surgical treatment of the coronary arteries, including angioplasty and the placement of stents, may be considered to keep the vessels open.

Heart failure. Heart failure can be the result of an enlarged, weakened heart, which has a hard time pumping enough blood to meet your body's needs (see pages 46-47). Or, the pumping may be normal, but a thickening of the pumping chamber on the left side of the heart doesn't permit normal expansion and relaxation of the muscle (diastolic heart failure). In some cases, this can cause fluid to build up in your lungs or your feet and legs.

For this reason, your doctor will target a lower blood pressure so that your heart won't have to work as hard. In fact, the most remarkable benefit of well-controlled high blood pressure is that it can lower your risk of developing heart failure by over 50 percent.

ACE inhibitors, ARBs and diuretics may be prescribed if you have heart failure in addition to high blood pressure. ACE inhibitors and ARBs reduce blood pressure by dilating your blood vessels, without interfering with your heart's pumping action. Diuretics reduce fluid buildup. The potassium-sparing diuretics spironolactone and eplerenone — which block aldosterone — have been shown to have lifesaving benefits in people with heart failure.

In most cases a beta blocker also may be appropriate. If you don't tolerate ACE inhibitors, an alternative option such as an ARB may be prescribed. Depending on your circumstances, you may choose to see a heart failure specialist because treatment programs are complex and a heart transplant may need to be considered.

High cholesterol. Many people with high blood pressure also have high cholesterol. Because having both conditions increases your risk of heart attack and stroke, you'll receive additional benefits from being able to lower both cholesterol and blood pressure.

The same lifestyle changes that help lower blood pressure can also help lower cholesterol levels. However, many people with high cholesterol may also need a cholesterol-lowering medication. Several studies suggest that statins, a class of drugs often prescribed to lower cholesterol, also seem to help lower systolic blood pressure but more research is needed to confirm these results.

As for blood pressure medications, don't take high doses of thiazide and loop diuretics if you also have high cholesterol. They can increase your cholesterol level and your triglycerides, another type of blood fat. Low doses of these drugs, though, don't produce the same effects. Beta blockers also may slightly raise your cholesterol. Should you need to take high doses of a beta blocker, having a good diet and taking cholesterol medication can help counteract the cholesterol increase.

Medications most often prescribed if you have high blood pressure and high cholesterol are ACE inhibitors, ARBs, calcium channel blockers, alpha blockers, central-acting agents and low-dose diuretics. A drug combining a calcium channel blocker and a statin also may be available with appropriate dosage of the individual drugs.

It's also important to avoid eating Seville (sour) oranges, pomelos, grapefruit, and drinking grapefruit juice if you're taking a cholesterol-lowering statin. That's because an interaction between the juice of these fruits and the statin can lead to a drug buildup in your blood. The same is true for some calcium channel blockers, so ask your doctor what he or she recommends.

Stroke and transient ischemic attack.
High blood pressure increases your risk of stroke and transient ischemic attack (TIA). If you're older than 55 and have a high pulse pressure, you may be at greater risk. At the age of 55 with normal blood pressure, the lifetime risk of stroke is one in five for women and one in six for men. This risk is double in people with high blood pressure (see pages 35-36).

Thrombolytic therapy can help reduce the effects of an ischemic stroke if it's given within the first hours after the onset of symptoms. The clot-busting (thrombolytic) drug is injected into your arteries to dissolve a blood clot — a common cause of stroke. If you think that you have symptoms of a stroke, including sudden numbness in your face, arm or leg, difficulty speaking, and sudden dizziness, seek emergency medical treatment immediately.

If you've had a stroke or TIA, your doctor may start you on a diuretic and an ACE inhibitor to help reduce your risk of a second stroke. ARBs and calcium channel blockers also may be prescribed. Using these drugs to lower blood pressure can reduce the risk of another stroke even if you've never had high blood pressure. One study

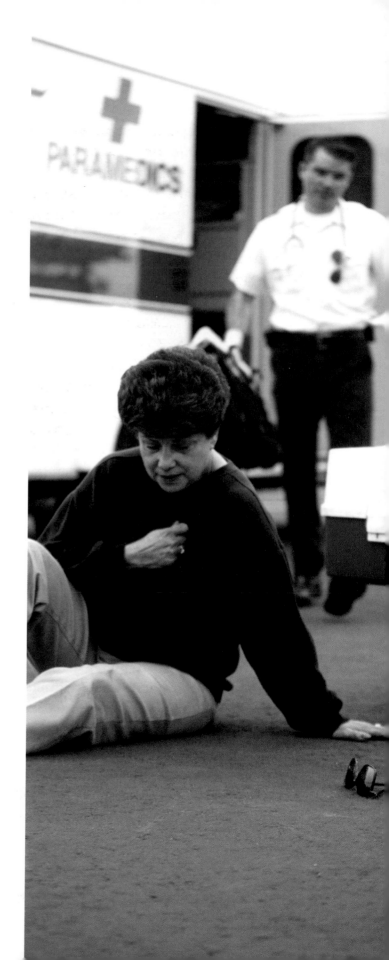

Not all experts agree on the definition of metabolic syndrome or whether it even exists as a distinct medical condition. Doctors have talked about this collection of risk factors for years and have called it many names, including syndrome X and insulin resistance syndrome. Whatever it's called, and however it's defined, the syndrome is apparently becoming more prevalent.

Diabetes

Diabetes and high blood pressure have a close association. About two-thirds of adults with diabetes have high blood pressure and, conversely, people with untreated high blood pressure have a higher incidence of diabetes. Having both conditions is a serious concern.

Many of the complications associated with diabetes can be attributed to having high blood pressure. High blood pressure also increases your chances of death from diabetes. A combination of high blood pressure, diabetes, high cholesterol and tobacco use puts you at extremely high risk of heart attack.

Aim for excellent control of your blood pressure, blood sugar (glucose) and blood fats. If you have diabetes and high blood pressure, you want to reduce your blood pressure to 130/80 mm Hg or lower. If you also have kidney disease, your doctor may recommend setting an even lower goal.

Lifestyle changes can help reduce your risk of serious complications from both diabetes and high blood pressure: Eat a healthy diet, get regular physical activity, limit your use of alcohol, and if you smoke or chew tobacco, stop doing so.

People who also have high cholesterol respond well to aggressive management. Lifestyle changes can reduce the risk by half of developing diabetes if you have prediabetes, impaired fasting glucose or obesity.

Medical therapy usually consists of ACE inhibitors or ARBs. They help protect your kidneys, which are at a higher risk of damage if you have both diseases. These drugs also have relatively few side effects.

Diuretics, beta blockers and calcium channel blockers also may be used to lower blood pressure and to prolong life. Alpha blockers are generally recommended last because they may strengthen orthostatic hypertension, a problem in some people with diabetes, and increase the risk of heart failure.

Often, combination drug therapy is needed to reach your target goal. If you're taking diuretics, your doctor will aim to keep your blood levels of potassium in the normal range — through diet or supplements — to reduce the likelihood of new-onset diabetes. If your blood pressure is controlled, daily aspirin is often advised.

Sleep apnea

Obstructive sleep apnea is a disorder in which breathing stops and starts repeatedly during sleep. It's relatively common in people with high blood pressure, particularly in people with a difficult-to-control form. Daytime drowsiness, snoring and prolonged pauses in breathing while sleeping are clues that the condition may be present. Obstructed airways as well as disturbances in the way your brain controls breathing can cause sleep apnea.

Although obesity is a risk factor for both hypertension and sleep apnea, recent studies suggest that sleep apnea independently contributes to hypertension, whether a person is obese or not. One theory centers on the fact that when your breathing stops during sleep, these pauses activate sympathetic nerve pathways — the part of your

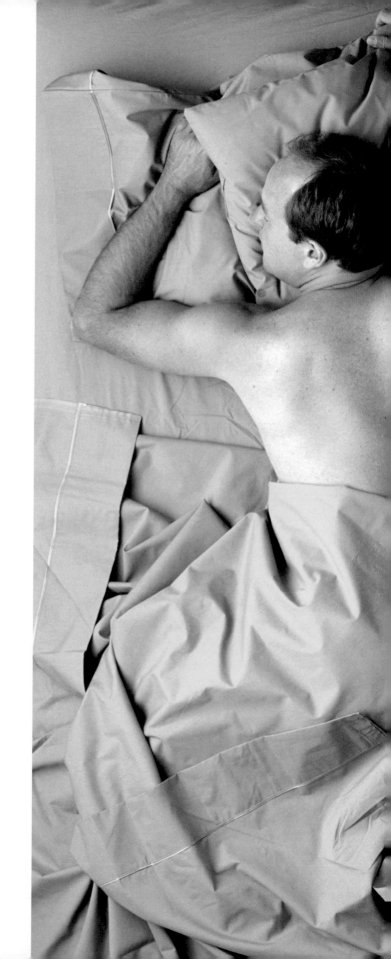

nervous system that prepares your body to react to stress or danger.

Activating this system "wakes up" your body so that you can start breathing again. The exaggerated activation of this system, such as occurs in people with sleep apnea, may result in a sustained increase in blood pressure.

More studies need to be done on the relationship between sleep apnea and hypertension. It's likely that treating sleep apnea — with continuous positive airway pressure (CPAP) therapy, weight loss and regular exercise — will improve daytime and nighttime blood pressure, as well, and decrease your risk of cardiovascular disease.

Kidney disease

Your kidneys play a vital role in removing extra fluid and waste from your body. This helps keep your blood pressure under control. But if the blood vessels in your kidneys are damaged from high blood pressure, the organs may become less efficient. This allows excess fluid to remain in your circulatory system, making high blood pressure worse. In turn, high blood pressure further weakens your kidneys, creating a dangerous cycle.

Most people with chronic kidney disease also have high blood pressure. The more impaired the kidneys are, the greater the risk of coronary artery disease, which is a common cause of disability and death among people who have chronic kidney disease.

Eventually, high blood pressure can lead to kidney (renal) failure, a condition in which your kidneys no longer function. In this end stage, life must be sustained with kidney dialysis or kidney transplant.

If you have kidney and cardiovascular disease as the result of high blood pressure, you'll need medications and lifestyle changes to prevent further damage to your kidneys and cardiovascular system. Blacks in America are more likely than whites to develop kidney problems from high blood pressure. Early treatment of hypertension is the best option for preventing the kidney problems from ever occurring.

If you have high blood pressure and kidney disease, the goal is to reduce your blood pressure to below 130/80 mm Hg, or lower if you have severe kidney disease. Once your blood pressure is lowered, the decline in kidney function also slows. If you have advanced kidney failure, you'll likely have special dietary needs that are best discussed with a dietitian.

Reduced sodium in your diet is important because impaired kidney function increases the level of sodium and fluids in your body. Diuretics also help flush out excess fluid. ACE inhibitors and ARBs are often the best medications for preventing further damage to your kidneys, and may be combined with a diuretic. However, they need to be used with caution due to potential side effects, such as too much potassium in your blood (hyperkalemia). Multiple drugs are usually required to reach a blood pressure goal.

A potentially reversible cause of kidney failure is the narrowing of the main artery leading to one or both kidneys (see pages 48-49). Atherosclerosis is the most common cause. Your doctor may consider widening the narrowed artery through angioplasty, stenting or surgery if your response to aggressive drug therapy is inadequate.

Sexual dysfunction

Some evidence indicates that sexual dysfunction is higher among people with uncontrolled high blood pressure.

Additional risk factors are similar to those for heart disease: diabetes, abnormal blood fats, obesity and lack of physical activity.

In men, erectile dysfunction (ED) is more likely in those with untreated high blood pressure than in those who take medication. Diuretics also may be associated with ED. Beta blockers haven't been associated with ED any more than other antihypertensive drugs, but it likely varies with the type of beta blocker used.

Although sexual dysfunction hasn't been studied as extensively in women with high blood pressure as in men, a recent report found that sexual dysfunction in women increased with their age and the amount of time they had high blood pressure. Adequate control of high blood pressure decreased the prevalence of sexual dysfunction in the participants, although treatment with beta blockers tended to increase sexual dysfunction. ACE inhibitors and ARBs appear to be least problematic in this regard for women. Improving arousal and lubrication also helped.

Before starting a high blood pressure medication, don't hesitate to discuss your current sexual function with your doctor. Report any changes after beginning the medication. If there are problems, another medication may be available that doesn't interfere with sexual function. For men, a class of drugs that includes sildenafil (Viagra), tadalafil (Cialis) and vardenafil (Levitra) is generally an acceptable treatment for ED and high blood pressure. Ask your doctor if it's appropriate for you.

Difficult-to-control high blood pressure

What if you've been following your doctor's orders, watching your weight, getting exercise and taking your medication, but you still aren't able to lower your blood pressure?

It could be that you're among a small group of people with hypertension whose blood pressure is resistant, or refractory — which means it doesn't fully respond to treatment. Resistant high blood pressure is defined as blood pressure that can't be brought below 140/90 mm Hg (or 130/80 mm Hg if you have diabetes, heart disease or kidney disease) using a combination of three different types of medication, including a diuretic.

It's rare for medications not to lower high blood pressure to the targeted goal in your treatment program. Often, it just takes time and trials with different drugs and doses to find the combination that works best.

If your medication isn't working, many times the first step is to try a different type of drug or a different combination of drugs in a single medication. Some medications simply work better for some people than for others.

The next step may be to add another medication to the one you're already taking, perhaps even a third or — if you have diabetes, heart disease or kidney failure and have lower blood pressure goals — even a fourth drug. Medications working in combination often have more powerful effects on your blood pressure than they would if you took them separately.

Rarely does anyone start out taking three different medications for high blood pressure, but sometimes this approach may be necessary — especially if your blood pressure goal is less

Are your blood pressure readings misleading?

In rare cases, resistant high blood pressure may be the result of a mistake in your diagnosis. Several factors can make your blood pressure appear higher than it actually is. They are:

- Pseudohypertension
- White-coat hypertension
- Blood pressure cuff size that's too small for your arm

See page 68 for more information on pseudohypertension and white-coat hypertension.

than 130/80 mm Hg. Common issues include inadequate diuretic therapy or the need for a more powerful diuretic, such as a loop diuretic.

Often, resistant high blood pressure stems from not making the lifestyle changes necessary to lower hypertension. If your blood pressure hasn't responded to drug therapy, ask yourself the following questions:

- *Have I been taking my medication exactly as prescribed?* Take your medication exactly as your doctor has ordered, or it may not work. If you think the pills cost too much or you find the regimen too hard to follow, talk to your doctor. Less expensive medications that you take only once a day can often be found.

- *Am I telling my doctor about all of the drugs and herbs I take?* Many medications and supplements, including over-the-counter products, may interfere with blood pressure medication. They include nonsteroidal anti-inflammatory drugs (NSAIDs), steroid medications, cold medicines, ephedra-like compounds, and herbs such as yohimbe.

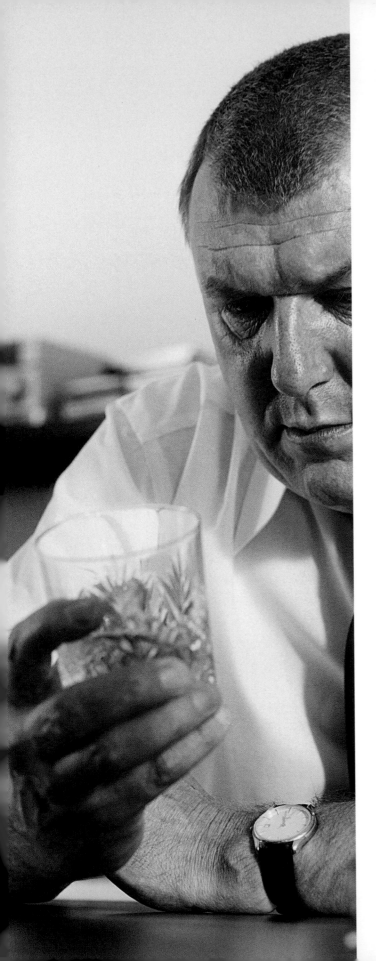

- *Have I cut down on sodium?* This doesn't mean table salt alone. Even if you aren't salting your foods, you may be eating processed foods with too much sodium. Read package labels to determine how much sodium is contained in a serving.
- *Am I drinking too much alcohol?* Alcohol can keep your blood pressure elevated, especially if you consume large amounts within a short time. Your medication may not be enough to overcome the effects of alcohol, and the alcohol may interfere with the action of the drug.
- *Have I seriously tried to stop smoking?* Like alcohol, tobacco products can keep blood pressure persistently high if you use them frequently.
- *Have I gained weight?* Generally, losing weight decreases your blood pressure. Weight gain — as few as 10 pounds — can increase it and make it harder to control.
- *Have I been sleeping well?* Sleep apnea can increase your blood pressure (see pages 245-246). The disorder occurs most frequently in older adults. Relieving the condition can reduce blood pressure.

If you, along with your doctor, have exhausted these possibilities, you still have other options. To begin with, you may need to consider stepping up the positive changes to your lifestyle. If you can walk another block, lose 1 more pound or make additional improvements in your diet, your high blood pressure may become less resistant to treatment. Reconsider the reversible causes of high blood pressure with your doctor, including medications for other conditions, certain supplements or foods, or conditions such as kidney abnormalities.

Your other options include adding a fourth drug to your daily regimen or increasing the dosage of your current medication. Aldosterone blockers in particular can play an important role in cases of resistant high blood pressure. The danger in increasing dosages is an increased risk of side effects from the medication. If you aren't already seeing a high blood pressure specialist, ask your doctor for a referral.

New treatments for resistant high blood pressure are being investigated, including a group of medications called endothelin antagonists and an implanted device that stimulates the carotid sinus, specialized parts of the carotid arteries in the neck that function in the regulation of heart rate and blood pressure.

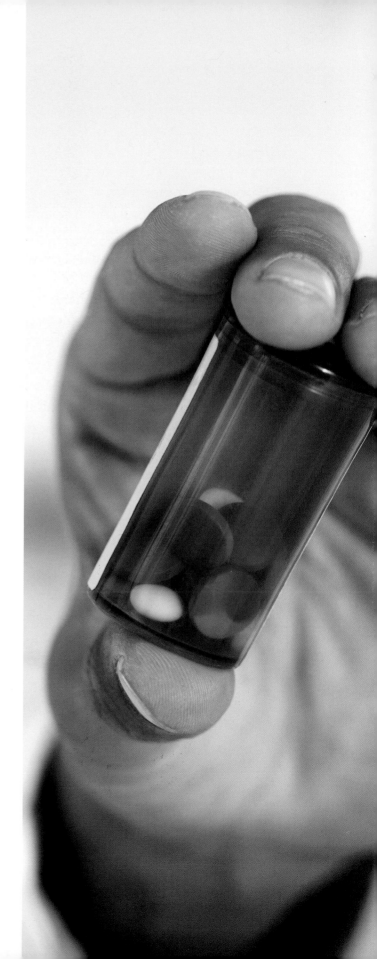

Wrap-up

Key points to remember
- Women and children have specific issues related to high blood pressure that merit special attention.
- High blood pressure during pregnancy must be monitored closely because of the risk, if left untreated, to the mother and to the baby.
- High blood pressure in children is often a sign of another health problem.
- High blood pressure in blacks appears more likely to develop at a younger age and result in more severe complications than for individuals in most other American ethnic groups.
- Aggressive treatment is necessary when high blood pressure is associated with another condition such as diabetes, high cholesterol, cardiovascular disease, stroke or kidney disease.
- Don't settle for poorly controlled hypertension. Work with your doctor to achieve your treatment goals.

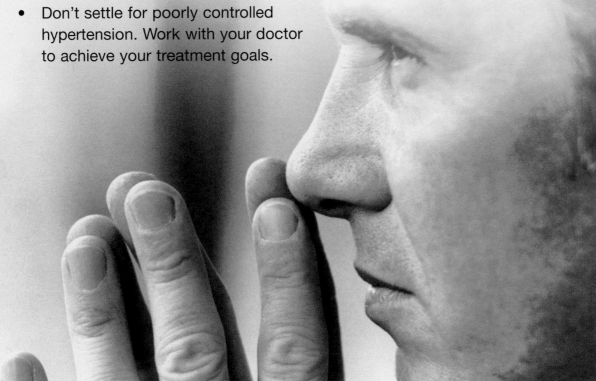

Glossary

aldosterone. A hormone secreted by the adrenal glands that regulates the balance of sodium and water in your body.

alpha blocker. A medication that blocks alpha receptors in the arteries, causing blood vessels to relax. It's typically prescribed in combination with other drugs.

angiotensin-converting enzyme (ACE) inhibitor. A medication that lowers blood pressure by disrupting the formation of angiotensin II.

angiotensin II. A substance that causes blood vessels to narrow (constrict) and stimulates the release of aldosterone.

angiotensin II receptor blocker (ARB). A blood pressure medication that blocks the action of angiotensin II in blood vessels. This drug affects angiotensin II at a different stage than the ACE inhibitor.

antihypertensives. A name for all the medications used to control high blood pressure.

aorta. The largest artery, which receives blood from the heart's left ventricle and supplies the other arteries in your circulatory system.

aortic valve. The valve between the left ventricle of the heart and aorta.

arrhythmia. Abnormal heartbeat.

arteriosclerosis. A condition in which the walls of arteries become hard and thick, sometimes interfering with the circulation of blood.

artery. A blood vessel that carries oxygenated blood from the heart to other tissues of the body.

atherosclerosis. A condition in which fatty deposits (plaques) accumulate in the interior lining of the arteries, resulting in narrowed pathways for blood to flow.

atria. Cavities or chambers, such as the two upper chambers of the heart that receive blood from veins. Singular form is atrium.

autonomic nervous system. Part of the the body's nervous system that controls involuntary actions. For example, it regulates heart rate and controls various glands.

B

beta blocker. A medication that limits the activity of epinephrine, a hormone that increases blood pressure and heart rate.

blood pressure. The force involved in keeping blood circulating continuously through your body. Pressure is placed on the inner walls of the arteries by the pumping action of the heart.

bruit. A French word used to describe the sound of turbulent blood flow, heard when a stethoscope is placed over a narrowed artery.

C

calcium channel blocker. A medication that lowers blood pressure by regulating calcium-related activity in the heart and blood vessels. Also called a calcium antagonist.

capillaries. Minute blood vessels connecting the smallest arteries to the smallest veins, forming intricate networks throughout the body.

cardiac. Relating to or situated near the heart.

cardiac cycle. The sequence of events taking place in the heart from the beginning of one heartbeat to the beginning of the next.

cardiac output. The volume of blood that the heart pumps through the circulatory system in one minute.

cardiology. The study of the heart and its function in good health and with disease.

cardiomyopathy. A muscle disorder that impairs the ability of the heart to pump blood.

cardiopulmonary. Relating to the heart and lungs.

cardiovascular. Relating to the heart and blood vessels.

cardiovascular system. The body system that provides a steady supply of oxygen-rich blood to cells and removes their waste. The system includes the heart, arteries, veins and the lymphatic system.

carotid arteries. The main arteries located in the neck that carry blood to the brain.

cholesterol. A lipid or fat-like substance found in the bloodstream and in body cells. People with high levels of cholesterol over a long period of time are at greater risk of heart disease.

circulatory system. Relating to the heart and blood vessels such as arteries and veins, and to the circulation of blood.

coronary. Relating to blood vessels of the heart.

coronary arteries. The arteries that supply blood to the heart.

coronary artery disease. The narrowing or blockage of one or more of the coronary arteries, resulting in decreased blood supply to the heart muscle.

D

diabetes. A chronic disease characterized by high levels of sugar (glucose) in the blood, often resulting in severe damage to the heart, blood vessels, kidneys and nerves.

diastole. A stage of the heart cycle in which the heart muscle relaxes, allowing blood to enter the ventricles (lower chambers) from the atria (upper chambers). From the ventricles, the blood will be pumped out of the heart and into the aorta.

diastolic pressure. The lowest blood pressure reached when the heart muscle relaxes. Listed as the second, or bottom, number in a blood pressure reading.

diuretic. A medication that increases the flow of urine out of the body. It's often used to treat conditions involving excess body fluids, such as high blood pressure and congestive heart failure.

E

edema. Swelling of body tissue due to the accumulation of excess fluid.

epinephrine. A naturally occurring hormone, also known as adrenaline, that helps prepare the body for danger or stress. It speeds up respiration and heart rate and increases blood pressure.

G

genetic. Relating to genes and to hereditary inheritance from parent to offspring.

glucose. A carbohydrate, also known as blood sugar, that's the body's main energy source.

H

HDL cholesterol. High-density lipoprotein cholesterol — the "good" cholesterol. A type of blood cholesterol thought to help protect against the accumulation of fatty deposits in blood vessels, which leads to atherosclerosis.

heart attack. An interruption in blood flow to the heart, causing the death of a part of the heart muscle. It's often due to blockage of one or more coronary arteries.

heart failure. A condition in which a weakened heart muscle is unable to pump enough blood to meet your body's needs.

heart rate. The number of contractions of the heart in one minute, which may vary according to how much oxygen you need.

heredity. The transmission of genetic traits from parent to offspring.

high blood pressure. A condition in which blood is pumped through the body under abnormally high pressure. Also called hypertension.

hyperkalemia. A condition caused by higher than normal levels of potassium in your blood.

hypernatremia. A condition caused by higher than normal levels of sodium in your blood.

hypertension. High blood pressure.

hypokalemia. A condition caused by lower than normal levels of potassium in your blood.

hyponatremia. A condition caused by lower than normal levels of sodium in your blood.

hypotension. Low blood pressure.

I

inferior vena cava. A large vein from the lower body that returns blood to the heart.

J

jugular veins. Veins in the neck that carry blood from the brain and head to the heart.

K

Korotkoff sounds. The sounds in an artery that are heard with a stethoscope as a blood pressure cuff is slowly deflated. These sounds help determine systolic and diastolic blood pressure.

L

LDL cholesterol. Low-density lipoprotein cholesterol — the "bad" cholesterol. A type of blood cholesterol that, in excess amounts, tends to accumulate along artery walls, obstructing blood flow.

lipid. A fat or fat-like substance in the bloodstream and in body cells, such as cholesterol.

M

metabolic syndrome. A cluster of disorders of your body's metabolism, including high blood pressure, elevated blood sugar levels, excess weight and high cholesterol levels.

mm Hg. An abbreviation for millimeters of mercury. Blood pressure is measured in these units.

myocardium. The muscular tissue layer in the wall of your heart.

N

noradrenaline. See norepinephrine.

norepinephrine. A naturally occurring hormone that's called into action when your body is under stress. This hormone increases heart rate and blood pressure and affects other body functions. Also called noradrenaline.

O

orthostatic hypotension. A significant drop in systolic blood pressure when an individual assumes a standing position. May cause dizziness, lightheadedness or fainting.

P

parasympathetic nervous system. A component of the autonomic nervous system that slows heart rate, relaxes the gastrointestinal tract and increases gland activity.

plaques. Deposits of fat cells and other substances in the inner lining of blood vessels, resulting in narrowed, less flexible arteries and obstructed blood flow.

potassium. An essential mineral that helps control heart rhythm. Also important to the nervous system and to muscle function.

preeclampsia. A condition that can occur in late pregnancy that's marked by high blood pressure and excess protein in urine.

pulmonary artery. A major blood vessel that carries oxygen-depleted blood from the heart to the lungs.

pulmonary veins. Several blood vessels that carry newly oxygenated blood from the lungs back to the heart.

pulse pressure. The difference between systolic blood pressure and diastolic blood pressure readings. A high pulse pressure may indicate increased risk of cardiovascular disease and stroke.

R

renin inhibitor. A medication that reduces the production of angiotensin II, a chemical that causes blood vessels to constrict.

risk factors. Factors that increase your chances of developing a disease or condition.

S

sodium. An essential mineral that helps maintain the proper fluid balance in your body.

sodium sensitivity. A response in certain individuals to their sodium intake, which can lead to higher blood pressure.

sphygmomanometer. A device used to measure systolic and diastolic blood pressure, which can be operated manually or electronically.

stethoscope. An instrument used for listening to sounds produced in the body, such as the sound of blood flowing through the arteries.

stroke. Damage to the brain caused by a disruption of blood flow, either from blockage of an artery or from a rupture in the artery wall.

superior vena cava. The large vein returning blood from the head and arms to the heart.

sympathetic nervous system. A component of the autonomic nervous system that increases heart rate, constricts blood vessels and reduces digestion.

systole. A stage of the heart cycle in which the heart muscle squeezes (contracts) to push blood out of the heart and into the aorta, followed by the diastole stage.

systolic pressure. The highest blood pressure produced by the contraction of the heart muscle during the systole stage. Listed as the first, or top, number in a blood pressure reading.

T

transient ischemic attack (TIA). A stroke-like event caused by temporary blockage of a blood vessel from something such as a blood clot. It differs from a stroke in that signs and symptoms generally disappear completely within 24 hours.

V

vascular. Relating to blood vessels.

vasodilator. A medication that widens (dilates) blood vessels.

vasopressor. A medication that increases blood pressure.

vein. A blood vessel that returns oxygen-depleted blood to the heart. Pressure in veins tends to be low.

venous. Relating to your veins.

ventricles. The two main pumping chambers of the heart, located below the atria. The left ventricle pumps oxygenated blood to the body, and the right ventricle pumps deoxygenated blood to the lungs.

Additional resources

Contact these organizations for more information about high blood pressure and associated conditions

American College of Cardiology
2400 N St. SW
Washington, DC 20037
202-375-6000
www.acc.org

American Diabetes Association
1701 N. Beauregard St.
Alexandria, VA 22311
800-342-2383
www.diabetes.org

American Heart Association
7272 Greenville Ave.
Dallas, TX 75231
800-242-8721
www.americanheart.org

American Society of Hypertension
148 Madison Ave., Fifth floor
New York, NY 10016
212-696-9099
www.ash-us.org

National Heart, Lung, and Blood Institute
P.O. Box 30105
Bethesda, MD 20824-0105
Recorded information:
800-575-9355
www.nhlbi.nih.gov

National Hypertension Association
324 East 30th St.
New York, NY 10016
212-889-3557
www.nathypertension.org

National Institute of Diabetes and Digestive and Kidney Diseases
Office of Communications and Public Liaison
NIDDK, National Institute of Health
31 Center Drive, MSC 2560
Bethesda, MD 20892-2560
800-438-5383
www2.niddk.nih.gov

National Kidney Foundation
30 East 33rd St.
New York, NY 10016
800-622-9010
www.kidney.org

National Stroke Association
9707 E. Easter Lane, Building B
Centennial, CO 80112
800-787-6537
www.stroke.org

World Hypertension League
100-1260 Hamilton Street
Suite 52
Vancouver, BC
Canada V6B 2S8
1-604-268-7176
www.worldhypertensionleague.org

Index

I

illicit drug
    interactions, 220
    use, 52, 71
illness, exercise and, 151–152
immunosuppressants, 53
inactivity, as risk factor, 42
injury avoidance, 148–152
    warning signs and, 151
    See also exercise
insulin resistance syndrome.
        See metabolic syndrome

J

jogging, 131–132
Joint National Committee on
    Prevention, Detection,
        Evaluation, and Treatment of
        High Blood Pressure, 77

K

kidney disease, 246–247
    medications, 246
    reduced sodium for, 247
    target blood pressure and, 54–55
    treatment goals and, 81
kidneys
    as blood pressure regulator, 23
    chronic failure, 46
    diuretics and, 186
    enlarged, 73
    imaging tests, 48
    polycystic, 48
    potassium and, 45
    renal artery obstruction, 48–49
    in secondary high blood pressure, 48
    in sodium regulation, 104

L

label reading, 117–119
left ventricle, 20, 21
left ventricular hypertrophy, 34–35

lifestyle changes
    for diabetes, 244
    goals, 82
    importance, 81
    for kidney disease, 246
    managing, 82
    for metabolic syndrome, 243
    for prehypertension, 80
    for resistant high blood pressure,
        249, 251
    for stress relief, 174–177
    as treatment, 77
    See also treatment
living with high blood pressure,
    205–226
    drug interactions, 215–224
    home monitoring, 206–213
    regular checkups, 213–215
low blood pressure, 30
lower back stretch, 142
lower carb approach, 89
lower sodium diets, 106–108
low potassium as risk factor, 45, 52

M

magnesium, 100
    sources, 103
    supplements, 101
    See also minerals
magnetic resonance angiography, 75
magnetic resonance imaging (MRI), 75
masked hypertension, 68
Mayo Clinic Healthy Weight Pyramid,
    89–90
meat and poultry, 97
    salt and, 112
    spice suggestions, 110
medical history, 69–71
    in healthy weight determination, 59
medication costs, reducing, 221–224
medications, 77
    herbal supplements and, 53
    over-the-counter (OTC), 52, 71, 160
    physical activity and, 136
    prescription, 53